KOKORO

BY

LAFCADIO HEARN

THE papers composing this volume treat of the inner rather than of the outer life of Japan,—for which reason they have been grouped under the title Kokoro (heart). Written with the above character, this word signifies also mind, in the emotional sense; spirit; courage; resolve; sentiment; affection; and inner meaning,—just as we say in English, "the heart of things."

KOBE September 15, 1895.

CONTENTS

I. AT A RAILWAY STATION
II. THE GENIUS Of JAPANESE CIVILIZATION
III. A STREET SINGER
IV. FROM A TRAVELING DIARY
V. THE NUN OF THE TEMPLE OF AMIDA
VI. AFTER THE WAR
VII. HARU
VIII. A GLIMPSE OF TENDENCIES
IX. BY FORCE OF KARMA
X. A CONSERVATIVE
XI. IN THE TWILIGHT OF THE GODS
XII. THE IDEA OF PRE-EXISTENCE

XIII. IN CHOLERA-TIME
XIV. SOME THOUGHTS ABOUT ANCESTOR-WORSHIP
XV. KIMIKO
APPENDIX. THREE POPULAR BALLADS

KOKORO

I

AT A RAILWAY STATION

Seventh day of the sixth Month;— twenty-sixth of Meiji.

Yesterday a telegram from Fukuoka announced that a desperate criminal captured there would be brought for trial to Kumamoto to-day, on the train due at noon. A Kumamoto policeman had gone to Fukuoka to take the prisoner in charge.

Four years ago a strong thief entered some house by night in the Street of the Wrestlers, terrified and bound the inmates, and carried away a number of valuable things. Tracked skillfully by the police, he was captured within twenty-four hours,—even before he could dispose of his plunder. But as he was being taken to the police station he burst his bonds, snatched the sword of his captor, killed him, and escaped. Nothing more was heard of him until last week.

Then a Kumamoto detective, happening to visit the Fukuoka prison, saw among the toilers a face that had been four years photographed upon his brain. "Who is that man?" he asked the guard. "A thief," was the reply, —"registered here as Kusabe." The detective walked up to the prisoner and said:—

"Kusabe is not your name. Nomura Teichi, you are needed in Kumamoto for murder." The felon confessed all.

I went with a great throng of people to witness the arrival at the station. I expected to hear and see anger; I even feared possibilities of violence. The murdered officer had been much liked; his relatives would certainly be among the spectators; and a Kumamoto crowd is not very gentle. I also thought to find many police on duty. My anticipations were wrong.

The train halted in the usual scene of hurry and noise,—scurry and clatter of passengers wearing geta,—screaming of boys wanting to sell Japanese newspapers and Kumamoto lemonade. Outside the barrier we waited for nearly five minutes. Then, pushed through the wicket by a police-sergeant, the prisoner appeared,—a large wild-looking man, with head bowed down, and arms fastened behind his back. Prisoner and guard both halted in front of the wicket; and the people pressed forward to see—but in silence. Then the officer called out,—

"Sugihara San! Sugihara O-Kibi! is she present?"

A slight small woman standing near me, with a child on her back, answered, "Hai!" and advanced through the press. This was the widow of the murdered man; the child she carried was his son. At a wave of the officer's hand the crowd fell back, so as to leave a clear space about the prisoner and his escort. In that space the woman with the child stood facing the murderer. The hush was of death.

Not to the woman at all, but to the child only, did the officer then speak. He spoke low, but so clearly that I could catch every syllable:—

"Little one, this is the man who killed your father four years ago. You had not yet been born; you were in your mother's womb. That you have no father to love you now is the doing of this man. Look at him—[here the officer, putting a hand to the prisoner's chin, sternly forced him to lift his eyes]—look well at him, little boy! Do not be afraid. It is painful; but it is your duty. Look at him!"

Over the mother's shoulder the boy gazed with eyes widely open, as in fear; then he began to sob; then tears came; but steadily and obediently he still looked—looked—looked—straight into the cringing face.

The crowd seemed to have stopped breathing.

I saw the prisoner's features distort; I saw him suddenly dash himself down upon his knees despite his fetters, and beat his face into the dust, crying out the while in a passion of hoarse remorse that made one's heart shake:—

"Pardon! pardon! pardon me, little one! That I did—not for hate was it done, but in mad fear only, in my desire to escape. Very, very wicked have I been; great unspeakable wrong have I done you! But now for my sin I go to die. I wish to die; I am glad to die! Therefore, O little one, be pitiful!—forgive me!"

The child still cried silently. The officer raised the shaking criminal; the dumb crowd parted left and right to let them by. Then, quite suddenly, the whole multitude began to sob. And as the bronzed guardian passed, I saw what I had never seen before, —what few men ever see,—what I shall probably never see again, —the tears of a Japanese policeman.

The crowd ebbed, and left me musing on the strange morality of the spectacle. Here was justice unswerving yet compassionate,— forcing knowledge of a crime by the pathetic witness of its simplest result. Here was desperate remorse, praying only for pardon before death. And here was a populace—perhaps the most dangerous in the Empire when angered—comprehending all, touched by all, satisfied with the contrition and the shame, and filled, not with wrath, but only with the great sorrow of the sin,—through simple deep experience of the difficulties of life and the weaknesses of human nature.

But the most significant, because the most Oriental, fact of the episode was that the appeal to remorse had been made through the criminal's sense of fatherhood,—that potential love of children which is so large a part of the soul of every Japanese.

There is a story that the most famous of all Japanese robbers, Ishikawa Goemon, once by night entering a house to kill and steal, was charmed by the smile of a baby which reached out hands to him, and that he remained playing with the little creature until all chance of carrying out his purpose was lost.

It is not hard to believe this story. Every year the police records tell of compassion shown to children by professional criminals. Some months ago a terrible murder case was reported in the local papers,—the slaughter of a household by robbers. Seven persons had been literally hewn to pieces while asleep; but the police discovered a little boy quite unharmed, crying alone in a pool of blood; and they found evidence unmistakable that the men who slew must have taken great care not to hurt the child.

II

THE GENIUS OF JAPANESE CIVILIZATION

I

Without losing a single ship or a single battle, Japan has broken down the power of China, made a new Korea, enlarged her own territory, and changed the whole political face of the East. Astonishing as this has seemed politically, it is much more astonishing psychologically; for it represents the result of a vast play of capacities with which the race had never been credited abroad,—capacities of a very high order. The psychologist knows that the so-called "adoption of Western civilization" within a time of thirty years cannot mean the addition to the Japanese brain of any organs or powers previously absent from it. He knows that it cannot mean any sudden change in the mental or moral character of the race. Such changes are not made in a generation. Transmitted civilization works much more slowly, requiring even hundreds of years to produce certain permanent psychological results.

It is in this light that Japan appears the most extraordinary country in the world; and the most wonderful thing in the whole episode of her "Occidentalization" is that the race brain could bear so heavy a shock. Nevertheless, though the fact be unique in human history, what does it really mean? Nothing more than rearrangement of a part of the pre-existing machinery of thought. Even that, for thousands of brave young minds, was death. The adoption of Western civilization was not nearly such an easy matter as un-thinking persons imagined. And it is quite evident that the mental readjustments, effected at a cost which remains to be told, have given good results only along directions in which the race had always shown capacities of special kinds. Thus, the appliances of Western industrial invention have worked admirably in Japanese hands,—have produced excellent results in those crafts at which the nation had been skillful, in other and quainter ways, for ages. There has been no transformation,

—nothing more than the turning of old abilities into new and larger channels. The scientific professions tell the same story. For certain forms of science, such as medicine, surgery (there are no better surgeons in the world than the Japanese), chemistry, microscopy, the Japanese genius is naturally adapted; and in all these it has done work already heard of round the world. In war and statecraft it has shown wonderful power; but throughout their history the Japanese have been characterized by great military and political capacity. Nothing remarkable has been done, however, in directions foreign to the national genius. In the study, for example, of Western music, Western art, Western literature, time would seem to have been simply wasted(1). These things make appeal extraordinary to emotional life with us; they make no such appeal to Japanese emotional life. Every serious thinker knows that emotional transformation of the individual through education is impossible. To imagine that the emotional character of an Oriental race could be transformed in the short space of thirty years, by the contact of Occidental ideas, is absurd. Emotional life, which is older than intellectual life, and deeper, can no more be altered suddenly by a change of milieu than the surface of a mirror can be changed by passing reflections. All that Japan has been able to do so miraculously well has been done without any self-transformation; and those who imagine her emotionally closer to us to-day than she may have been thirty years ago ignore facts of science which admit of no argument.

Sympathy is limited by comprehension. We may sympathize to the same degree that we understand. One may imagine that he sympathizes with a Japanese or a Chinese; but the sympathy can never be real to more than a small extent outside of the simplest phases of common emotional life,— those phases in which child and man are at one. The more complex feelings of the Oriental have been composed by combinations of experiences, ancestral and individual, which have had no really precise correspondence in Western life, and which we can therefore not fully know. For converse reasons, the Japanese cannot, even though they would, give Europeans their best sympathy.

But while it remains impossible for the man of the West to discern the true color of Japanese life, either intellectual or emotional (since the one is woven into the other), it is equally impossible for him to escape the conviction that, compared with his own, it is very small. It is dainty; it holds delicate potentialities of rarest interest and value; but it is otherwise so small that Western life, by contrast with it, seems almost supernatural. For we must judge visible and measurable manifestations. So judging, what a contrast between the emotional and intellectual worlds of West and East! Far less striking that between the frail wooden streets of the Japanese capital and the tremendous solidity of a thoroughfare in Paris or London. When one compares the utterances which West and East have given to their dreams, their aspirations, their sensations,—a Gothic cathedral with a Shinto temple, an opera by Verdi or a trilogy by Wagner with a performance of geisha, a European epic with a Japanese poem,—how incalculable the difference in emotional volume, in imaginative power, in artistic synthesis! True, our music is an essentially modern art; but in looking back through all our past the difference in creative force is scarcely less marked,—not surely in the period of Roman magnificence, of marble amphitheatres and of aqueducts spanning provinces, nor in the Greek period of the divine in sculpture and of the supreme in literature.

And this leads to the subject of another wonderful fact in the sudden development of Japanese power. Where are the outward material signs of that immense new force she has been showing both in productivity and in war? Nowhere! That which we miss in her emotional and intellectual life is missing also from her industrial and commercial life,—largeness! The land remains what it was before; its face has scarcely been modified by all the changes of Meiji. The miniature railways and telegraph poles, the bridges and tunnels, might almost escape notice in the ancient green of the landscapes. In all the cities, with the exception of the open ports and their little foreign settlements, there exists hardly a street vista suggesting the teaching of Western ideas. You might journey two hundred miles through the interior of the country, looking in vain for large manifestations of the new civilization. In no place do you find commerce exhibiting its ambition in gigantic warehouses, or industry expanding its machinery under acres of roofing. A Japanese city is still, as it was ten centuries ago, little more than a wilderness of wooden sheds,—picturesque, indeed, as paper lanterns are, but scarcely less frail. And there is no great stir and noise anywhere,—no heavy traffic, no booming and rumbling, no furious haste. In Tokyo itself you may enjoy, if you wish, the peace of a country village. This want of visible or audible signs of the new-found force which is now menacing the markets of the West and changing the maps of the far East gives one a queer, I might even say a weird feeling. It is almost the sensation received when, after climbing through miles of silence to reach some Shinto shrine, you find voidness only and solitude,—an elfish, empty little wooden structure, mouldering in shadows a thousand years old. The strength of Japan, like the strength of her ancient faith, needs little material display: both exist where the deepest real power of any great people exists,—in the Race Ghost.

(1) In one limited sense, Western art has influenced Japanese. literature and drama; but the character of the influence proves the racial difference to which I refer. European plays have been reshaped for the Japanese stage, and European novels rewritten for Japanese readers. But a literal version is rarely attempted; for the original incidents, thoughts, and emotions would be unintelligible to the average reader or playgoer. Plots are adopted; sentiments and incidents are totally transformed. "The New Magdalen" becomes a Japanese girl who married an Eta. Victor Hugo's *Les Miserables*

becomes a tale of the Japanese civil war; and Enjolras a Japanese student. There have been a few rare exceptions, including the marked success of a literal translation of the *Sorrows of Werther*.

II

As I muse, the remembrance of a great city comes back to me,—a city walled up to the sky and roaring like the sea. The memory of that roar returns first; then the vision defines: a chasm, which is a street, between mountains, which are houses. I am tired, because I have walked many miles between those precipices of masonry, and have trodden no earth,—only slabs of rock,—and have heard nothing but thunder of tumult. Deep below those huge pavements I know there is a cavernous world tremendous: systems underlying systems of ways contrived for water and steam and fire. On either hand tower facades pierced by scores of tiers of windows,—cliffs of architecture shutting out the sun. Above, the pale blue streak of sky is cut by a maze of spidery lines,—an infinite cobweb of electric wires. In that block on the right there dwell nine thousand souls; the tenants of the edifice facing it pay the annual rent of a million dollars. Seven millions scarcely covered the cost of those bulks overshadowing the square beyond,—and there are miles of such. Stairways of steel and cement, of brass and stone, with costliest balustrades, ascend through the decades and double-decades of stories; but no foot treads them. By water-power, by steam, by electricity, men go up and down; the heights are too dizzy, the distances too great, for the use of the limbs. My friend who pays rent of five thousand dollars for his rooms in the fourteenth story of a monstrosity not far off has never trodden his stairway. I am walking for curiosity alone; with a serious purpose I should not walk: the spaces are too broad, the time is too precious, for such slow exertion,—men travel from district to district, from house to office, by steam. Heights are too great for the voice to traverse; orders are given and obeyed by machinery. By electricity far-away doors are opened; with one touch a hundred rooms are lighted or heated.

And all this enormity is hard, grim, dumb; it is the enormity of mathematical power applied to utilitarian ends of solidity and durability. These leagues of palaces, of warehouses, of business structures, of buildings describable and indescribable, are not beautiful, but sinister. One feels depressed by the mere sensation of the enormous life which created them, life without sympathy; of their prodigious manifestation of power, power without pity. They are the architectural utterance of the new industrial age. And there is no halt in the thunder of wheels, in the storming of hoofs and of human feet. To ask a question, one must shout into the ear of the questioned; to see, to understand, to move in that high-pressure medium, needs experience. The unaccustomed feels the sensation of being in a panic, in a tempest, in a cyclone. Yet all this is order.

The monster streets leap rivers, span sea-ways, with bridges of stone, bridges of steel. Far as the eye can reach, a bewilderment of masts, a web-work of rigging, conceals the shores, which are cliffs of masonry. Trees in a forest stand less thickly, branches in a forest mingle less closely, than the masts and spars of that immeasurable maze. Yet all is order.

III

Generally speaking, we construct for endurance, the Japanese for impermanency. Few things for common use are made in Japan with a view to durability. The straw sandals worn out and replaced at each stage of a journey, the robe consisting of a few simple widths loosely stitched together for wearing, and unstitched again for washing, the fresh chopsticks served to each new guest at a hotel, the light shoji frames serving at once for windows and walls, and repapered twice a year; the mattings renewed every autumn,—all these are but random examples of countless small things in daily life that illustrate the national contentment with impermanency.

What is the story of a common Japanese dwelling? Leaving my home in the morning, I observe, as I pass the corner of the next street crossing mine, some men setting up bamboo poles on a vacant lot there. Returning after five hours' absence, I find on the same lot the skeleton of a two-story house. Next forenoon I see that the walls are nearly finished already,—mud and wattles. By sundown the roof has been completely tiled. On the following morning I observe that the mattings have been put down, and the inside plastering has been finished. In five days the house is completed. This, of course, is a cheap building; a fine one would take much longer to put up and finish. But Japanese cities are for the most part composed of such common buildings. They are as cheap as they are simple.

I cannot now remember where I first met with the observation that the curve of the Chinese roof might preserve the memory of the nomad tent. The idea haunted me long after I had ungratefully forgotten the book in which I found it; and when I first saw, in Izumo, the singular structure of the old Shinto temples, with queer cross-projections at their gable-ends and upon their roof-ridges, the suggestion of the forgotten essayist about the possible origin of much less ancient forms returned to me with great force. But there is much in Japan besides primitive architectural traditions to indicate a nomadic ancestry for the race. Always and everywhere there is a total absence of what we would call solidity; and the characteristics of impermanence seem to mark almost everything in the exterior life of the people, except, indeed, the immemorial costume of the peasant and the shape of the implements of his toil. Not to dwell upon the fact that even during the comparatively brief period of her written history Japan has had more than sixty capitals, of which the greater number have completely disappeared, it may be broadly stated that every Japanese city is rebuilt within the time of a generation. Some temples and a few colossal fortresses offer exceptions; but, as a general rule, the Japanese city changes its substance, if not its form, in the lifetime of a man. Fires, earth-quakes, and many other causes partly account for this; the chief reason, however, is that houses are not built to last. The common people have no ancestral homes. The dearest spot to all is, not the place of birth, but the place of burial; and there is little that is permanent save the resting-places of the dead and the sites of the ancient shrines.

The land itself is a land of impermanence. Rivers shift their courses, coasts their outline, plains their level; volcanic peaks heighten or crumble; valleys are blocked by lava-floods or landslides; lakes appear and disappear. Even the matchless shape of Fuji, that snowy miracle which has been the inspiration of artists for centuries, is said to have been slightly changed since my advent to the country; and not a few other mountains have in the same short time taken totally new forms. Only the general lines of the land, the general aspects of its nature, the general character of the seasons, remain fixed. Even the very beauty of the landscapes is largely illusive,—a beauty of shifting colors and moving mists. Only he to whom those landscapes are familiar can know how their mountain vapors make mockery of real changes which have been, and ghostly predictions of other changes yet to be, in the history of the archipelago.

The gods, indeed, remain,—haunt their homes upon the hills, diffuse a soft religious awe through the twilight of their groves, perhaps because they are without form and substance. Their shrines seldom pass utterly into oblivion, like the dwellings of men. But every Shinto temple is necessarily rebuilt at more or less brief intervals; and the holiest,—the shrine of Ise,— in obedience to immemorial custom, must be demolished every twenty years, and its timbers cut into thousands of tiny charms, which are distributed to pilgrims.

From Aryan India, through China, came Buddhism, with its vast doctrine of impermanency. The builders of the first Buddhist temples in Japan—architects of another race—built well: witness the Chinese structures at Kamakura that have survived so many centuries, while of the great city which once surrounded them not a trace remains. But the psychical influence of Buddhism could in no land impel minds to the love of material stability. The teaching that the universe is an illusion; that life is but one momentary halt upon an infinite journey; that all attachment to persons, to places, or to things must be fraught with sorrow; that only through suppression of every desire—even the desire of Nirvana itself—can humanity reach the eternal peace, certainly harmonized with the older racial feeling. Though the people never much occupied themselves with the profounder philosophy of the foreign faith, its doctrine of impermanency must, in course of time, have profoundly influenced national character. It explained and consoled; it imparted new capacity to bear all things bravely; it strengthened that patience which is a trait of the race. Even in Japanese art—developed, if not actually created, under Buddhist influence—the doctrine of impermanency has left its traces. Buddhism taught that nature was a dream, an illusion, a phantasmagoria; but it also taught men how to seize the fleeting impressions of that dream, and how to interpret them in relation to the highest truth. And they learned well. In the flushed splendor of the blossom-bursts of spring, in the coming and the going of the cicada, in the dying crimson of autumn foliage, in the ghostly beauty of snow, in the delusive motion of wave or cloud, they saw old parables of perpetual meaning. Even their calamities—fire, flood, earthquake, pestilence—interpreted to them unceasingly the doctrine of the eternal Vanishing.

All things which exist in Time must perish. The forests, the mountains,—all things thus exist. In Time are born all things having desire.

The Sun and Moon, Sakra himself with all the multitude of his attendants, will all, without exception, perish; there is not one that will endure.

In the beginning things were fixed; in the end again they separate: different combinations cause other substance; for in nature there is no uniform and constant principle.

All component things must grow old; impermanent are all component things. Even unto a grain of sesamum seed there is no such thing as a compound which is permanent. All are transient; all have the inherent quality of dissolution.

All component things, without exception, are impermanent, unstable, despicable, sure to depart, disintegrating; all are temporary as a mirage, as a phantom, or as foam…. Even as all earthen vessels made by the potter end in being broken, so end the lives of men.

And a belief in matter itself is unmentionable and inexpressible,—it is neither a thing nor no-thing: and this is known even by children and ignorant persons.

IV

Now it is worth while to inquire if there be not some compensatory value attaching to this impermanency and this smallness in the national life.

Nothing is more characteristic of that life than its extreme fluidity. The Japanese population represents a medium whose particles are in perpetual circulation. The motion is in itself peculiar. It is larger and more eccentric than the motion of Occidental populations, though feebler between points. It is also much more natural,—so natural that it could not exist in Western civilization. The relative mobility of a European population and the Japanese population might be expressed by a comparison between certain high velocities of vibration and certain low ones. But the high velocities would represent, in such a comparison, the consequence of artificial force applied; the slower vibrations would not. And this difference of kind would mean more than surface indications could announce. In one sense, Americans may be right in thinking themselves great travelers. In another, they are certainly wrong; the man of the people in America cannot compare, as a traveler, with the man of the people in Japan. And of course, in considering relative mobility of populations, one must consider chiefly the great masses, the workers,—not merely the small class of wealth. In their own country, the Japanese are the greatest travelers of any civilized people. They are the greatest travelers because, even in a land composed mainly of mountain chains, they recognize no obstacles to travel. The Japanese who travels most is not the man who needs railways or steamers to carry him.

Now, with us, the common worker is incomparably less free than the common worker in Japan. He is less free because of the more complicated mechanism of Occidental societies, whose forces tend to agglomeration and solid integration. He is less free because the social and industrial machinery on which he must depend reshapes him to its own particular requirements, and always so as to evolve some special and artificial capacity at the cost of other inherent capacity. He is less free because he must live at a standard making it impossible for him to win financial independence by mere thrift. To achieve any such independence, he must possess exceptional character and exceptional faculties greater than those of thousands of exceptional competitors equally eager to escape from the same thralldom. In brief, then, he is less independent because the special character of his civilization numbs his natural power to live without the help of machinery or large capital. To live thus artificially means to lose, sooner or later, the power of independent movement. Before a Western man can move he has many things to consider. Before a Japanese moves he has nothing to consider. He simply leaves the place he dislikes, and goes to the place he wishes, without any trouble. There is nothing to prevent him. Poverty is not an obstacle, but a stimulus. Impedimenta he has none, or only such as he can dispose of in a few minutes. Distances have no significance for him. Nature has given him perfect feet that can spring him over fifty miles a day without pain; a stomach whose chemistry can extract ample nourishment from food on which no European could live; and a constitution that scorns heat, cold, and damp alike, because still unimpaired by unhealthy clothing, by superfluous comforts, by the habit of seeking warmth from grates and stoves, and by the habit of wearing leather shoes.

It seems to me that the character of our footgear signifies more than is commonly supposed. The footgear represents in itself a check upon individual freedom. It signifies this even in costliness; but in form it signifies infinitely more. It has distorted the Western foot out of the original shape, and rendered it incapable of the work for which it was evolved. The physical results are not limited to the foot. Whatever acts as a check, directly or indirectly, upon the organs of locomotion must extend its effects to the whole physical constitution. Does the evil stop even there? Perhaps we submit to conventions the most absurd of any existing in any civilization because we have too long submitted to the tyranny of shoemakers. There may be defects in our politics, in our social ethics, in our religious system, more or less related to the habit of wearing leather shoes. Submission to the cramping of the body must certainly aid in developing submission to the cramping of the mind.

The Japanese man of the people—the skilled laborer able to underbid without effort any Western artisan in the same line of industry—remains happily independent of both shoemakers and tailors. His feet are good to look at, his body is healthy, and his heart is free. If he desire to travel a thousand miles, he can get ready for his journey in five minutes. His whole outfit need not cost seventy-five cents; and all his baggage can be put into a handkerchief. On ten dollars he can travel for a year without work, or he can travel simply on his ability to work, or he can travel as a pilgrim. You may reply that any savage can do the same thing. Yes, but any civilized man cannot; and the Japanese has been a highly civilized man for at least a thousand years. Hence his present capacity to threaten Western manufacturers.

We have been too much accustomed to associate this kind of independent mobility with the life of our own beggars and tramps, to have any just conception of its intrinsic meaning. We have thought of it also in connection with unpleasant things,—uncleanliness and bad smells. But, as Professor Chamberlain has well said, "a Japanese crowd is the sweetest in the world" Your Japanese tramp takes his hot bath daily, if he has a fraction of a cent to pay for it, or his cold bath, if he has not. In his little bundle there are combs, toothpicks, razors, toothbrushes. He never allows himself to become unpleasant. Reaching his destination, he can transform himself into a visitor of very nice manners, and faultless though simple attire(1).

Ability to live without furniture, without impedimenta, with the least possible amount of neat clothing, shows more than the advantage held by this Japanese race in the struggle of life; it shows also the real character of some weaknesses in our own civilization. It forces reflection upon the useless multiplicity of our daily wants. We must have meat and bread and butter; glass windows and fire; hats, white shirts, and woolen underwear; boots and shoes; trunks, bags, and boxes; bedsteads, mattresses, sheets, and blankets: all of which a Japanese can do without, and is really better off without. Think for a moment how important an article of Occidental attire is the single costly item of white shirts! Yet even the linen shirt, the so-called "badge of a gentleman," is in itself a useless garment. It gives neither warmth nor comfort. It represents in our fashions the survival of something once a luxurious class distinction, but to-day meaningless and useless as the buttons sewn on the outside of coat-sleeves.

(1) Critics have tried to make fun of Sir Edwin Arnold's remark that a Japanese crowd smells like a geranium-flower. Yet the simile is exact! The perfume called jako, when sparingly used, might easily be taken for the odor of a musk-geranium. In almost any Japanese assembly including women a slight perfume of jako is discernible; for the robes worn have been laid in drawers containing a few grains of jako. Except for this delicate scent, a Japanese crowd is absolutely odorless.

V

The absence of any huge signs of the really huge things that Japan has done bears witness to the very peculiar way in which her civilization has been working. It cannot forever so work; but it has so worked thus far with amazing success. Japan is producing without capital, in our large sense of the word. She has become industrial without becoming essentially mechanical and artificial. The vast rice crop is raised upon millions of tiny, tiny farms; the silk crop, in millions of small poor homes, the tea crop, on countless little patches of soil. If you visit Kyoto to order something from one of the greatest porcelain makers in the world, one whose products are known better in London and in Paris than even in Japan, you will find the factory to be a wooden cottage in which no American farmer would live. The greatest maker of cloisonne vases, who may ask you two hundred dollars for something five inches high, produces his miracles behind a two-story frame dwelling containing perhaps six small rooms. The best girdles of silk made in Japan, and famous throughout the Empire, are woven in a house that cost scarcely five hundred dollars to build. The work is, of course, hand-woven. But the factories weaving by machinery—and weaving so well as to ruin foreign industries of far vaster capacity—are hardly more imposing, with very few exceptions. Long, light, low one-story or two-story sheds they are, about as costly to erect as a row of wooden stables with us. Yet sheds like these turn out silks that sell all round the world. Sometimes only by inquiry, or by the humming of the machinery, can you distinguish a factory from an old yashiki, or an old-fashioned Japanese school building,—unless indeed you can read the Chinese characters over the garden gate. Some big brick factories and breweries exist; but they are very few, and even when close to the foreign settlements they seem incongruities in the landscape.

Our own architectural monstrosities and our Babels of machinery have been brought into existence by vast integrations of industrial capital. But such integrations do not exist in the Far East; indeed, the capital to make them does not exist. And supposing that in the course of a few generations there should form in Japan corresponding combinations of money power, it is not easy to suppose correspondences in architectural construction. Even two-story edifices of brick have given bad results in the leading commercial centre; and earthquakes seem to condemn Japan to perpetual simplicity in building. The very land revolts against the imposition of Western architecture, and occasionally even opposes the new course of traffic by pushing railroad lines out of level and out of shape.

Not industry alone still remains thus unintegrated; government itself exhibits a like condition. Nothing is fixed except the Throne. Perpetual change is identical with state policy. Ministers, governors, superintendents, inspectors, all high civil and military officials, are shifted at irregular and surprisingly short intervals, and hosts of smaller officials scatter each time with the whirl. The province in which I passed the first twelvemonth of my residence in Japan has had four different governors in five years. During my stay at Kumamoto, and before the war had begun, the military command of that important post was three times changed. The government college had in three years three directors. In educational circles, especially, the rapidity of such changes has been phenomenal. There have been five different ministers of education in my own time, and more than five different educational policies. The twenty-six thousand public schools are so related in their management to the local assemblies that, even were no other influences at work, constant change would be inevitable because of the changes in the assemblies. Directors and teachers keep circling from post to post; there are men little more than thirty years old who have taught in almost every province of the country. That any educational system could have produced any great results under these conditions seems nothing short of miraculous.

We are accustomed to think that some degree of stability is necessary to all real progress, all great development. But Japan has given proof irrefutable that enormous development is possible without any stability at all. The explanation is in the race character,—a race character in more ways than one the very opposite of our own. Uniformly mobile, and thus uniformly impressionable, the nation has moved unitedly in the direction of great ends, submitting the whole volume of its forty millions to be moulded by the ideas of its rulers, even as sand or as water is shaped by wind. And this submissiveness to reshaping belongs to the old conditions of its soul life,—old conditions of rare unselfishness and perfect faith. The relative absence from the national character of egotistical individualism has been the saving of an empire; has enabled a great people to preserve its independence against prodigious odds. Wherefore Japan may well be grateful to her two great religions, the creators and the preservers of her moral power to Shinto, which taught the individual to think of his Emperor and of his country before thinking either of his own family or of himself; and to Buddhism, which trained him to master regret, to endure pain, and to accept as eternal law the vanishing of things loved and the tyranny of things hated.

To-day there is visible a tendency to hardening,—a danger of changes leading to the integration of just such an officialism as that which has proved the curse and the weakness of China. The moral results of the new education have not been worthy of the material results. The charge of want of "individuality," in the accepted sense of pure selfishness, will scarcely be made against the Japanese of the next century. Even the compositions of students already reflect the new conception of intellectual strength only as a weapon of offense, and the new sentiment of aggressive egotism. "Impermanency," writes one, with a fading memory of Buddhism in his mind, "is the nature of our life. We see often persons who were rich yesterday, and are poor to-day. This is the result of human competition, according to the law of evolution. We are exposed to that competition. We must fight each other, even if we are not inclined to do so. With what sword shall we fight? With the sword of knowledge, forged by education."

Well, there are two forms of the cultivation of Self. One leads to the exceptional development of the qualities which are noble, and the other signifies something about which the less said the better. But it is not the former which the New Japan is now beginning to study. I confess to being one of those who believe that the human heart, even in the history of a race, may be worth infinitely more than the human intellect, and that it will sooner or later prove itself infinitely better able to answer all the cruel enigmas of the Sphinx of Life. I still believe that the old Japanese were nearer to the solution of those enigmas than are we, just because they recognized moral beauty as greater than intellectual beauty. And, by way of conclusion, I may venture to quote from an article on education by Ferdinand Brunetiere:—

"All our educational measures will prove vain, if there be no effort to force into the mind, and to deeply impress upon it, the sense of those fine words of Lamennais: '*Human society is based upon mutual giving, or upon the sacrifice of man for man, or of each man for all other men; and sacrifice is the very essence of all true society.*' It is this that we have been unlearning for nearly a century; and if we have to put ourselves to school afresh, it will be in order that we may learn it again. Without such knowledge there can be no society and no education,—not, at least, if the object of education be to form man for society. Individualism is to-day the enemy of education, as it is also the enemy of social order. It has not been so always; but it has so become. It will not be so forever; but it is so now. And without striving to destroy it-which would mean to fall from one extreme into another—we must recognize that, no matter what we wish to do for the family, for society, for education, and for the country, it is against individualism that the work will have to be done."

III

A STREET SINGER

A woman carrying a samisen, and accompanied by a little boy seven or eight years old, came to my house to sing. She wore the dress of a peasant, and a blue towel tied round her head. She was ugly; and her natural ugliness had been increased by a cruel attack of smallpox. The child carried a bundle of printed ballads.

Neighbors then began to crowd into my front yard,—mostly young mothers and nurse girls with babies on their backs, but old women and men likewise—the inkyo of the vicinity. Also the jinrikisha-men came from their stand at the next street-corner; and presently there was no more room within the gate.

The woman sat down on my doorstep, tuned her samisen, played a bar of accompaniment,—and a spell descended upon the people; and they stared at each other in smiling amazement.

For out of those ugly disfigured lips there gushed and rippled a miracle of a voice—young, deep, unutterably touching in its penetrating sweetness. "Woman or wood-fairy?" queried a bystander. Woman only,—but a very, very great artist. The way she handled her instrument might have astounded the most skillful geisha; but no such voice had ever been heard from any geisha, and no such song. She sang as only a peasant can sing,—with vocal rhythms learned, perhaps, from the cicada and the wild nightingales,—and with fractions and semi-fractions and demi-semi-fractions of tones never written down in the musical language of the West.

And as she sang, those who listened began to weep silently. I did not distinguish the words; but I felt the sorrow and the sweetness and the patience of the life of Japan pass with her voice into my heart,—plaintively seeking for something never there. A tenderness invisible seemed to gather and quiver about us; and sensations of places and of times forgotten came softly back, mingled with feelings ghostlier,—feelings not of any place or time in living memory.

Then I saw that the singer was blind.

When the song was finished, we coaxed the woman into the house, and questioned her. Once she had been fairly well to do, and had learned the samisen when a girl. The little boy was her son. Her husband was paralyzed. Her eyes had been destroyed by smallpox. But she was strong, and able to walk great distances. When the child became tired, she would carry him on her back. She could support the little one, as well as the bed-ridden husband, because whenever she sang the people cried, and gave her coppers and food…. Such was her story. We gave her some money and a meal; and she went away, guided by her boy.

I bought a copy of the ballad, which was about a recent double suicide: "*The sorrowful ditty of Tamayone and Takejiro,— composed by Tabenaka Yone of Number Fourteen of the Fourth Ward of Nippon-bashi in the South District of the City of Osaka.*" It had evidently been printed from a wooden block; and there were two little pictures. One showed a girl and boy sorrowing together. The other—a sort of tail-piece—represented a writing-stand, a dying lamp, an open letter, incense burning in a cup, and a vase containing shikimi,—that sacred plant used in the Buddhist ceremony of making offerings to the dead. The queer cursive text, looking like shorthand written perpendicularly, yielded to translation only lines like these:—

"In the First Ward of Nichi-Hommachi, in far-famed Osaka— *O the sorrow of this tale of shinju!*

"Tamayone, aged nineteen,—to see her was to love her, for Takejiro, the young workman.

"For the time of two lives they exchange mutual vows— *O the sorrow of loving a courtesan!*

"On their arms they tattoo a Raindragon, and the character 'Bamboo'—thinking never of the troubles of life....

"But he cannot pay the fifty-five yen for her freedom— *O the anguish of Takejiro's heart!*

"Both then vow to pass away together, since never in this world can they become husband and wife....

"Trusting to her comrades for incense and for flowers— *O the pity of their passing like the dew!*

"Tamayone takes the wine-cup filled with water only, in which those about to die pledge each other....

"*O the tumult of the lovers' suicide!—O the pity of their lives thrown away!*"

In short, there was nothing very unusual in the story, and nothing at all remarkable in the verse. All the wonder of the performance had been in the voice of the woman. But long after the singer had gone that voice seemed still to stay,—making within me a sense of sweetness and of sadness so strange that I could not but try to explain to myself the secret of those magical tones.

And I thought that which is hereafter set down:—

All song, all melody, all music, means only some evolution of the primitive natural utterance of feeling,—of that untaught speech of sorrow, joy, or passion, whose words are tones. Even as other tongues vary, so varies this language of tone combinations. Wherefore melodies which move us deeply have no significance to Japanese ears; and melodies that touch us not at all make powerful appeal to the emotion of a race whose soul-life differs from our own as blue differs from yellow….Still, what is the reason of the deeper feelings evoked in me—an alien—by this Oriental chant that I could never even learn,—by this common song of a blind woman of the people? Surely that in the voice of the singer there were qualities able to make appeal to something larger than the sum of the experience of one race,—to something wide as human life, and ancient as the knowledge of good and evil.

One summer evening, twenty-five years ago, in a London park, I heard a girl say "Good-night" to somebody passing by. Nothing but those two little words,—"Good-night." Who she was I do not know: I never even saw her face; and I never heard that voice again. But still, after the passing of one hundred seasons, the memory of her "Good-night" brings a double thrill incomprehensible of pleasure and pain,—pain and pleasure, doubtless, not of me, not of my own existence, but of pre-existences and dead suns.

For that which makes the charm of a voice thus heard but once cannot be of this life. It is of lives innumerable and forgotten. Certainly there never have been two voices having precisely the same quality. But in the utterance of affection there is a tenderness of timbre common to the myriad million voices of all humanity. Inherited memory makes familiar to even the newly-born the meaning of the tone of caress. Inherited, no doubt, likewise, our knowledge of the tones of sympathy, of grief, of pity. And so the chant of a blind woman in this city of the Far East may revive in even a Western mind emotion deeper than individual being,—vague dumb pathos of forgotten sorrows,—dim loving impulses of generations unremembered. The dead die never utterly. They sleep in the darkest cells of tired hearts and busy brains,—to be startled at rarest moments only by the echo of some voice that recalls their past.

IV

FROM A TRAVELING DIARY

I

OSAKA-KYOTO RAILWAY.
April 15, 1895.

Feeling drowsy in a public conveyance, and not being able to lie down, a Japanese woman will lift her long sleeve before her face ere she begins to nod. In this second-class railway-carriage there are now three women asleep in a row, all with faces screened by the left sleeve, and all swaying together with the rocking of the train, like lotos-flowers in a soft current. (This use of the left sleeve is either fortuitous or instinctive; probably instinctive, as the right hand serves best to cling to strap or seat in case of shock.) The spectacle is at once pretty and funny, but especially pretty, as exemplifying that grace with which a refined Japanese woman does everything,—always in the daintiest and least selfish way possible. It is pathetic, too, for the attitude is also that of sorrow, and sometimes of weary prayer. All because of the trained sense of duty to show only one's happiest face to the world.

Which fact reminds me of an experience.

A male servant long in my house seemed to me the happiest of mortals. He laughed invariably when spoken to, looked always delighted while at work, appeared to know nothing of the small troubles of life. But one day I peeped at him when he thought himself quite alone, and his relaxed face startled me. It was not the face I had known. Hard lines of pain and anger appeared in it, making it seem twenty years older. I coughed gently to announce my presence. At once the face smoothed, softened, lighted up as by a miracle of rejuvenation. Miracle, indeed, of perpetual unselfish self-control.

II

Kyoto, April 16.

The wooden shutters before my little room in the hotel are pushed away; and the morning sun immediately paints upon my shoji, across squares of gold light, the perfect sharp shadow of a little peach-tree. No mortal artist—not even a Japanese—could surpass that silhouette! Limned in dark blue against the yellow glow, the marvelous image even shows stronger or fainter tones according to the varying distance of the unseen branches outside. it sets me thinking about the possible influence on Japanese art of the use of paper for house-lighting purposes.

By night a Japanese house with only its shoji closed looks like a great paper-sided lantern,—a magic-lantern making moving shadows within, instead of without itself. By day the shadows on the shoji are from outside only; but they may be very wonderful at the first rising of the sun, if his beams are leveled, as in this instance, across a space of quaint garden.

There is certainly nothing absurd in that old Greek story which finds the origin of art in the first untaught attempt to trace upon some wall the outline of a lover's shadow. Very possibly all sense of art, as well as all sense of the supernatural, had its simple beginnings in the study of shadows. But shadows on shoji are so remarkable as to suggest explanation of certain Japanese faculties of drawing by no means primitive, but developed beyond all parallel, and otherwise difficult to account for. Of course, the quality of Japanese paper, which takes shadows better than any frosted glass, must be considered, and also the character of the shadows themselves. Western vegetation, for example, could scarcely furnish silhouettes so gracious as those of Japanese garden-trees, all trained by centuries of caressing care to look as lovely as Nature allows.

I wish the paper of my shoji could have been, like a photographic plate, sensitive to that first delicious impression cast by a level sun. I am already regretting distortions: the beautiful silhouette has begun to lengthen.

III

Kyoto, April 16.

Of all peculiarly beautiful things in Japan, the most beautiful are the approaches to high places of worship or of rest,—the Ways that go to Nowhere and the Steps that lead to Nothing.

Certainly, their special charm is the charm of the adventitious, —the effect of man's handiwork in union with Nature's finest moods of light and form and color,—a charm which vanishes on rainy days; but it is none the less wonderful because fitful.

Perhaps the ascent begins with a sloping paved avenue, half a mile long, lined with giant trees. Stone monsters guard the way at regular intervals. Then you come to some great flight of steps ascending through green gloom to a terrace umbraged by older and vaster trees; and other steps from thence lead to other terraces, all in shadow. And you climb and climb and climb, till at last, beyond a gray torii, the goal appears: a small, void, colorless wooden shrine,—a Shinto miya. The shock of emptiness thus received, in the high silence and the shadows, after all the sublimity of the long approach, is very ghostliness itself.

Of similar Buddhist experiences whole multitudes wait for those who care to seek them. I might suggest, for example, a visit to the grounds of Higashi Otani, which are in the city of Kyoto. A grand avenue leads to the court of a temple, and from the court a flight of steps fully fifty feet wide—massy, mossed, and magnificently balustraded—leads to a walled terrace. The scene makes one think of the approach to some Italian pleasure-garden of Decameron days. But, reaching the terrace, you find only a gate, opening—into a cemetery! Did the Buddhist landscape-gardener wish to tell us that all pomp and power and beauty lead only to such silence at last?

IV

KYOTO, April 10-20.

I have passed the greater part of three days in the national Exhibition,—time barely sufficient to discern the general character and significance of the display. It is essentially industrial, but nearly all delightful, notwithstanding, because of the wondrous application of art to all varieties of production. Foreign merchants and keener observers than I find in it other and sinister meaning,—the most formidable menace to Occidental trade and industry ever made by the Orient. "Compared with England," wrote a correspondent of the London Times, "it is farthings for pennies throughout.... The story of the Japanese invasion of Lancashire is older than that of the invasion of Korea and China. It has been a conquest of peace,—a painless process of depletion which is virtually achieved.... The Kyoto display is proof of a further immense development of industrial enterprise.... A country where laborers' hire is three shillings a week, with all other domestic charges in proportion, must—other things being equal—kill competitors whose expenses are quadruple the Japanese scale." Certainly the industrial jiujutsu promises unexpected results.

The price of admission to the Exhibition is a significant matter also. Only five sen! Yet even at this figure an immense sum is likely to be realized,—so great is the swarm of visitors. Multitudes of peasants are pouring daily into the city,—pedestrians mostly, just as for a pilgrimage. And a pilgrimage for myriads the journey really is, because of the inauguration festival of the greatest of Shinshu temples.

The art department proper I thought much inferior to that of the Tokyo Exhibition of 1890. Fine things there were, but few. Evidence, perhaps, of the eagerness with which the nation is turning all its energies and talents in directions where money is to be made; for in those larger departments where art is combined with industry,—such as ceramics, enamels, inlaid work, embroideries,—no finer and costlier work could ever have been shown. Indeed, the high value of certain articles on display suggested a reply to a Japanese friend who observed, thoughtfully, "If China adopts Western industrial methods, she will be able to underbid us in all the markets of the world."

"Perhaps in cheap production," I made answer. "But there is no reason why Japan should depend wholly upon cheapness of production. I think she may rely more securely upon her superiority in art and good taste. The art-genius of a people may have a special value against which all competition by cheap labor is vain. Among Western nations, France offers an example. Her wealth is not due to her ability to underbid her neighbors. Her goods are the dearest in the world: she deals in things of luxury and beauty. But they sell in all civilized countries because they are the best of their kind. Why should not Japan become the France of the Further East?"

The weakest part of the art display is that devoted to oil-painting,—oil-painting in the European manner. No reason exists why the Japanese should not be able to paint wonderfully in oil by following their own particular methods of artistic expression. But their attempts to follow Western methods have even risen to mediocrity only in studies requiring very realistic treatment. Ideal work in oil, according to Western canons of art, is still out of their reach. Perhaps they may yet discover for themselves a new gateway to the beautiful, even through oil-painting, by adaptation of the method to the particular needs of the race-genius; but there is yet no sign of such a tendency.

A canvas representing a perfectly naked woman looking at herself in a very large mirror created a disagreeable impression. The Japanese press had been requesting the removal of the piece, and uttering comments not flattering to Western art ideas. Nevertheless the canvas was by a Japanese painter. It was a daub; but it had been boldly priced at three thousand dollars.

I stood near the painting for a while to observe its effect upon the people, —peasants by a huge majority. They would stare at it, laugh scornfully, utter some contemptuous phrase, and turn away to examine the kakemono, which were really far more worthy of notice though offered at prices ranging only from ten to fifty yen. The comments were chiefly leveled at "foreign" ideas of good taste (the figure having been painted with a European head). None seemed to consider the thing as a Japanese work. Had it represented a Japanese woman, I doubt whether the crowd would have even tolerated its existence.

Now all this scorn for the picture itself was just. There was nothing ideal in the work. It was simply the representation of a naked woman doing what no woman could like to be seen doing. And a picture of a mere naked woman, however well executed, is never art if art means idealism. The realism of the thing was its offensiveness. Ideal nakedness may be divine,—the most godly of all human dreams of the superhuman. But a naked person is not divine at all. Ideal nudity needs no girdle, because the charm is of lines too beautiful to be veiled or broken. The living real human body has no such divine geometry. Question: Is an artist justified in creating nakedness for its own sake, unless he can divest that nakedness of every trace of the real and personal?

There is a Buddhist text which truly declares that he alone is wise who can see things without their individuality. And it is this Buddhist way of seeing which makes the greatness of the true Japanese art.

V

These thoughts came:—

That nudity which is divine, which is the abstract of beauty absolute, gives to the beholder a shock of astonishment and delight,—not unmixed with melancholy. Very few works of art give this, because very few approach perfection. But there are marbles and gems which give it, and certain fine studies of them, such as the engravings published by the Society of Dilettanti. The longer one looks, the more the wonder grows, since there appears no line, or part of a line, whose beauty does not surpass all remembrance. So the secret of such art was long thought supernatural; and, in very truth, the sense of beauty it communicates is more than human,—is superhuman, in the meaning of that which is outside of existing life,—is therefore supernatural as any sensation known to man can be.

What is the shock?

It resembles strangely, and is certainly akin to, that psychical shock which comes with the first experience of love. Plato explained the shock of beauty as being the Soul's sudden half-remembrance of the World of Divine

Ideas. "They who see here any image or resemblance of the things which are there receive a shock like a thunderbolt, and are, after a manner, taken out of themselves." Schopenhauer explained, the shock of first love as the Willpower of the Soul of the Race. The positive psychology of Spencer declares in our own day that the most powerful of human passions, when it makes its first appearance, is absolutely antecedent to all individual experience. Thus do ancient thought and modern—metaphysics and science—accord in recognizing that the first deep sensation of human beauty known to the individual is not individual at all.

Must not the same truth hold of that shock which supreme art gives? The human ideal expressed in such art appeals surely to the experience of all that Past enshrined in the emotional life of the beholder,—to something inherited from innumerable ancestors.

Innumerable indeed!

Allowing three generations to a century, and presupposing no consanguineous marriages, a French mathematician estimates that each existing individual of his nation would have in his veins the blood of twenty millions of contemporaries of the year 1000. Or calculating from the first year of our own era, the ancestry of a man of to-day would represent a total of eighteen quintillions. Yet what are twenty centuries to the time of the life of man!

Well, the emotion of beauty, like all of our emotions, is certainly the inherited product of unimaginably countless experiences in an immeasurable past. In every aesthetic sensation is the stirring of trillions of trillions of ghostly memories buried in the magical soil of the brain. And each man carries within him an ideal of beauty which is but an infinite composite of dead perceptions of form, color, grace, once dear to look upon. It is dormant, this ideal,—potential in essence,—cannot be evoked at will before the imagination; but it may light up electrically at any perception by the living outer senses of some vague affinity. Then is felt that weird, sad, delicious thrill, which accompanies the sudden backward-flowing of the tides of life and time; then are the sensations of a million years and of myriad generations summed into the emotional feeling of a moment.

Now, the artists of one civilization only—the Greeks—were able to perform the miracle of disengaging the Race-Ideal of beauty from their own souls, and fixing its wavering out-line in jewel and stone. Nudity, they made divine; and they still compel us to feel its divinity almost as they felt it themselves. Perhaps they could do this because, as Emerson suggested, they possessed all-perfect senses. Certainly it was not because they were as beautiful as their own statues. No man and no woman could be that. This only is sure,—that they discerned and clearly fixed their ideal,—composite of countless million remembrances of dead grace in eyes and eyelids, throat and cheek, mouth and chin, body and limbs.

The Greek marble itself gives proof that there is no absolute individuality,—that the mind is as much a composite of souls as the body is of cells.

VI

Kyoto, April 21.

The noblest examples of religious architecture in the whole empire have just been completed; and the great City of Temples is now enriched by two constructions probably never surpassed in all the ten centuries of its existence. One is the gift of the Imperial Government; the other, the gift of the common people.

The government's gift is the Dai-Kioku-Den,—erected to commemorate the great festival of Kwammu Tenno, fifty-first emperor of Japan, and founder of the Sacred City. To the Spirit of this Emperor the Dai-Kioku-Den is dedicated: it is thus a Shinto temple, and the most superb of all Shinto temples. Nevertheless, it is not Shinto architecture, but a facsimile of the original palace of Kwammu Tenno upon the original scale. The effect upon national sentiment of this magnificent deviation from conventional forms, and the profound poetry of the reverential feeling which suggested it, can be fully comprehended only by those who know that Japan is still practically ruled by the dead. Much more than beautiful are the edifices of the Dai-Kioku-Den. Even in this most archaic of Japan cities they startle; they tell to the sky in every tilted line of their horned roofs the tale of another and more fantastic age. The most eccentrically striking parts of the whole are the two-storied and five-towered gates,—veritable Chinese dreams, one would say. In color the construction is not less oddly attractive than in form,—and this especially because of the fine use made of antique green tiles in the polychromatic roofing. Surely the august Spirit of Kwammu Tenno might well rejoice in this charming evocation of the past by architectural necromancy!

But the gift of the people to Kyoto is still grander. It is represented by the glorious Higashi Hongwanji,—or eastern Hongwan temple (Shinshu). Western readers may form some idea of its character from the simple statement that it cost eight millions of dollars and required seventeen years to build. In mere dimension it is largely exceeded by other Japanese buildings of cheaper construction; but anybody familiar with the Buddhist

VII

Kobe, April 23.

I have been visiting the exhibition of fishes and of fisheries which is at Hyogo, in a garden by the sea. Waraku-en is its name, which signifies, "The Garden of the Pleasure of Peace." It is laid out like a landscape garden of old time, and deserves its name. Over its verge you behold the great bay, and fishermen in boats, and the white far-gliding of sails splendid with light, and beyond all, shutting out the horizon, a lofty beautiful massing of peaks mauve-colored by distance.

I saw ponds of curious shapes, filled with clear sea-water, in which fish of beautiful colors were swimming. I went to the aquarium where stranger kinds of fishes swam behind glass—fishes shaped like toy-kites, and fishes shaped like sword-blades, and fishes that seemed to turn themselves inside out, and funny, pretty fishes of butterfly-colors, that move like dancing-girls, waving sleeve-shaped fins.

I saw models of all manner of boats and nets and hooks and fish-traps and torch-baskets for night-fishing. I saw pictures of every kind of fishing, and both models and pictures of men killing whales. One picture was terrible,—the death agony of a whale caught in a giant net, and the leaping of boats in a turmoil of red foam, and one naked man on the monstrous back—a single figure against the sky—striking with a great steel, and the fountain-gush of blood responding to the stroke.... Beside me I heard a Japanese father and mother explain the picture to their little boy; and the mother said:—

"When the whale is going to die, it speaks; it cries to the Lord Buddha for help,—*Namu Amida Butsu!*"

I went to another part of the garden where there were tame deer, and a "golden bear" in a cage, and peafowl in an aviary, and an ape. The people fed the deer and the bear with cakes, and tried to coax the peacock to open its tail, and grievously tormented the ape. I sat down to rest on the veranda of a pleasure-house near the aviary, and the Japanese folk who had been looking at the picture of whale-fishing found their way to the same veranda; and presently I heard the little boy say:—

"Father, there is an old, old fisherman in his boat. Why does he not go to the Palace of the Dragon-King of the Sea, like Urashima?"

The father answered: "Urashima caught a turtle which was not really a turtle, but the Daughter of the Dragon-King. So he was rewarded for his kindness. But that old fisherman has not caught any turtle, and even if he had caught one, he is much too old to marry. Therefore he will not go to the Palace."

Then the boy looked at the flowers, and the fountains, and the sunned sea with its white sails, and the mauve-colored mountains beyond all, and exclaimed:—

"Father, do you think there is any place more beautiful than this in the whole world?"

The father smiled deliciously, and seemed about to answer, but before he could speak the child cried out, and leaped, and clapped his little hands for delight, because the peacock had suddenly outspread the splendor of its tail. And all hastened to the aviary. So I never heard the reply to that pretty question.

But afterwards I thought that it might have been answered thus:—

"My boy, very beautiful this is. But the world is full of beauty; and there may be gardens more beautiful than this.

"But the fairest of gardens is not in our world. It is the Garden of Amida, in the Paradise of the West.

"And whosoever does no wrong what time he lives may after death dwell in that Garden.

"There the divine Kujaku, bird of heaven, sings of the Seven Steps and the Five Powers, spreading its tail as a sun.

"There lakes of jewel-water are, and in them lotos-flowers of a loveliness for which there is not any name. And from those flowers proceed continually rays of rainbow-light, and spirits of Buddhas newly-born.

"And the water, murmuring among the lotos-buds, speaks to the souls in them of Infinite Memory and Infinite Vision, and of the Four Infinite Feelings.

"And in that place there is no difference between gods and men, save that under the splendor of Amida even the gods must bend; and all sing the hymn of praise beginning, '*O Thou of Immeasurable Light!*'

"But the Voice of the River Celestial chants forever, like the chanting of thousands in unison: '*Even this is not high; there is still a Higher! This is not real; this is not Peace!*'"

V

THE NUN OF THE TEMPLE OF AMIDA

When O-Toyo's husband—a distant cousin, adopted into her family for love's sake—had been summoned by his lord to the capital, she did not feel anxious about the future. She felt sad only. It was the first time since their bridal that they had ever been separated. But she had her father and mother to keep her company, and, dearer than either,—though she would never have confessed it even to herself,—her little son. Besides, she always had plenty to do. There were many household duties to perform, and there was much clothing to be woven—both silk and cotton.

Once daily at a fixed hour, she would set for the absent husband, in his favorite room, little repasts faultlessly served on dainty lacquered trays,— miniature meals such as are offered to the ghosts of the ancestors, and to the gods(1). These repasts were served at the east side of the room, and his kneeling-cushion placed before them. The reason they were served at the east side, was because he had gone east. Before removing the food, she always lifted the cover of the little soup-bowl to see if there was vapor upon its lacquered inside surface. For it is said that if there be vapor on the inside of the lid covering food so offered, the absent beloved is well. But if there be none, he is dead,—because that is a sign that his soul has returned by itself to seek nourishment. O-Toyo found the lacquer thickly beaded with vapor day by day.

The child was her constant delight. He was three years old, and fond of asking questions to which none but the gods know the real answers. When he wanted to play, she laid aside her work to play with him. When he wanted to rest, she told him wonderful stories, or gave pretty pious answers to his questions about those things which no man can ever understand. At evening, when the little lamps had been lighted before the holy tablets and the images, she taught his lips to shape the words of filial prayer. When he had been laid to sleep, she brought her work near him, and watched the still sweetness of his face. Sometimes he would smile in his dreams; and she knew that Kwannon the divine was playing shadowy play with him, and she would murmur the Buddhist invocation to that Maid "who looketh forever down above the sound of prayer."

Sometimes, in the season of very clear days, she would climb the mountain of Dakeyama, carrying her little boy on her back. Such a trip delighted him much, not only because of what his mother taught him to see, but also of what she taught him to hear. The sloping way was through groves and woods, and over grassed slopes, and around queer rocks; and there were flowers with stories in their hearts, and trees holding tree-spirits. Pigeons cried korup-korup; and doves sobbed owao, owao and cicada wheezed and fluted and tinkled.

All those who wait for absent dear ones make, if they can, a pilgrimage to the peak called Dakeyama. It is visible from any part of the city; and from its summit several provinces can be seen. At the very top is a stone of almost human height and shape, perpendicularly set up; and little pebbles are heaped before it and upon it. And near by there is a small Shinto shrine erected to the spirit of a princess of other days. For she mourned the absence of one she loved, and used to watch from this mountain for his coming until she pined away and was changed into a stone. The people therefore built the shrine; and lovers of the absent still pray there for the return of those dear to them; and each, after so praying, takes home one of the little pebbles heaped there. And when the beloved one returns, the pebble must be taken back to the pebble-pile upon the mountain-top, and other pebbles with it, for a thank-offering and commemoration.

Always ere O-Toyo and her son could reach their home after such a day, the dusk would fall softly about them; for the way was long, and they had to both go and return by boat through the wilderness of rice-fields round the town,—which is a slow manner of journeying. Sometimes stars and fireflies lighted them; sometimes also the moon,—and O-Toyo would softly sing to her boy the Izumo child-song to the moon:—

   Nono-San,
Little Lady Moon,
How old are you?
"Thirteen days,—
Thirteen and nine."
That is still young,
And the reason must be
For that bright red obi,
So nicely tied(2),
And that nice white girdle
About your hips.
Will you give it to the horse?
"Oh, no, no!"
Will you give it to the cow?
"Oh, no, no!(3)"

And up to the blue night would rise from all those wet leagues of labored field that great soft bubbling chorus which seems the very voice of the soil itself,—the chant of the frogs. And O-Toyo would interpret its syllables to the child: Me kayui! me kayui! "Mine eyes tickle; I want to sleep."

All those were happy hours.

(1) Such a repast, offered to the spirit of the absent one loved, is called a Kage-zen; lit., "Shadow-tray." The word zen is also use to signify the meal served on the lacquered tray,—which has feet, like miniature table. So that time term "Shadow-feast" would be a better translation of Kage-zen.

(2) Because an obi or girdle of very bright color can be worn only by children.

(3) Nono-San,
or
O-Tsuki-san
Ikutsu?
"Jiu-san,—
Kokonotsu."

Sore wa mada
Wakai yo,
Wakai ye mo
Dori
Akai iro no
Obi to,
Shire iro no
Obi to
Koshi ni shanto
Musun de.
Uma ni yaru?
"Iyaiya!"
Ushi ni yaru?
"Iyaiya!"

II

Then twice, within the time of three days, those masters of life and death whose ways belong to the eternal mysteries struck at her heart. First she was taught that the gentle husband for whom she had so often prayed never could return to her,—having been returned unto that dust out of which all forms are borrowed. And in another little while she knew her boy slept so deep a sleep that the Chinese physician could not waken him. These things she learned only as shapes are learned in lightning flashes. Between and beyond the flashes was that absolute darkness which is the pity of the gods.

It passed; and she rose to meet a foe whose name is Memory. Before all others she could keep her face, as in other days, sweet and smiling. But when alone with this visitant, she found herself less strong. She would arrange little toys and spread out little dresses on the matting, and look at them, and talk to them in whispers, and smile silently. But the smile would ever end in a burst of wild, loud weeping; and she would beat her head upon the floor, and ask foolish questions of the gods.

One day she thought of a weird consolation,—that rite the people name Toritsu-banashi,—the evocation of the dead. Could she not call back her boy for one brief minute only? It would trouble the little soul; but would he not gladly bear a moment's pain for her dear sake? Surely!

[To have the dead called back one must go to some priest—Buddhist or Shinto—who knows the rite of incantation. And the mortuary tablet, or ihai, of the dead must be brought to that priest.

Then ceremonies of purification are performed; candles are lighted and incense is kindled before the ihai; and prayers or parts of sutras are recited; and offerings of flowers and of rice are made. But, in this case, the rice must not be cooked. And when everything has been made ready, the priest, taking in his left hand an instrument shaped like a bow, and striking it rapidly with his right, calls upon the name of the dead, and cries out the words, Kitazo yo! kitazo yo! kitazo yo! meaning, "I have come(1)." And, as he cries, the tone of his voice gradually changes until it becomes the very voice of the dead person,—for the ghost enters into him.

Then the dead will answer questions quickly asked, but will cry continually: "Hasten, hasten! for this my coming back is painful, and I have but a little time to stay!" And having answered, the ghost passes; and the priest falls senseless upon his face.

Now to call back the dead is not good. For by calling them back their condition is made worse. Returning to the underworld, they must take a place lower than that which they held before.

To-day these rites are not allowed by law. They once consoled; but the law is a good law, and just,—since there exist men willing to mock the divine which is in human hearts.]

So it came to pass that O-Toyo found herself one night in a lonely little temple at the verge of the city,—kneeling before the ihai of her boy, and hearing the rite of incantation. And presently, out of the lips of the officiant there came a voice she thought she knew,—a voice loved above all others, —but faint and very thin, like a sobbing of wind.

And the thin voice cried to her:—

"Ask quickly, quickly, mother! Dark is the way and long; and I may not linger."

Then tremblingly she questioned:—

"Why must I sorrow for my child? What is the justice of the gods?"

And there was answer given:—

"O mother, do not mourn me thus! That I died was only that you might not die. For the year was a year of sickness and of sorrow,—and it was given me to know that you were to die; and I obtained by prayer that I should take your place(2).

"O mother, never weep for me! it is not kindness to mourn for the dead. Over the River of Tears(3) their silent road is; and when mothers weep, the flood of that river rises, and the soul cannot pass, but must wander to and fro.

"Therefore, I pray you, do not grieve, O mother mine! Only give me a little water sometimes."

(1) Whence the Izumo saying about one who too often announces his coming: "Thy talk is like the talk of necromancy!"—Toritsubanashi no yona.

(2) Migawari, "substitute," is the religious term.

(3) "Namida-no-Kawa."

III

From that hour she was not seen to weep. She performed, lightly and silently, as in former days, the gentle duties of a daughter.

Seasons passed; and her father thought to find another husband for her. To the mother, he said:—

"If our daughter again have a son, it will be great joy for her, and for all of us."

But the wiser mother made answer:—

"Unhappy she is not. It is impossible that she marry again. She has become as a little child, knowing nothing of trouble or sin."

It was true that she had ceased to know real pain. She had begun to show a strange fondness for very small things. At first she had found her bed too large—perhaps through the sense of emptiness left by the loss of her child; then, day by day, other things seemed to grow too large,—the dwelling itself, the familiar rooms, the alcove and its great flower-vases,—even the household utensils. She wished to eat her rice with miniature chop-sticks out of a very small bowl such as children use.

In these things she was lovingly humored; and in other matters she was not fantastic. The old people consulted together about her constantly. At last the father said:—

"For our daughter to live with strangers might be painful. But as we are aged, we may soon have to leave her. Perhaps we could provide for her by making her a nun. We might build a little temple for her."

Next day the mother asked O-Toyo:—

"Would you not like to become a holy nun, and to live in a very, very small temple, with a very small altar, and little images of the Buddhas? We should be always near you. If you wish this, we shall get a priest to teach you the sutras."

O-Toyo wished it, and asked that an extremely small nun's dress be got for her. But the mother said:—

"Everything except the dress a good nun may have made small. But she must wear a large dress—that is the law of Buddha."

So she was persuaded to wear the same dress as other nuns.

IV

They built for her a small An-dera, or Nun's-Temple, in an empty court where another and larger temple, called Amida-ji, had once stood. The An-dera was also called Amida-ji, and was dedicated to Amida-Nyorai and to other Buddhas. It was fitted up with a very small altar and with miniature altar furniture. There was a tiny copy of the sutras on a tiny reading-desk, and tiny screens and bells and kakemono. And she dwelt there long after her parents had passed away. People called her the Amida-ji no Bikuni,— which means The Nun of the Temple of Amida.

A little outside the gate there was a statue of Jizo. This Jizo was a special Jizo—the friend of sick children. There were nearly always offerings of small rice-cakes to be seen before him. These signified that some sick child was being prayed for; and the number of the rice-cakes signified the number of the years of the child. Most often there were but two or three cakes; rarely there were seven or ten. The Amida-ji no Bikuni took care of the statue, and supplied it with incense-offerings, and flowers from the temple garden; for there was a small garden behind the An-dera.

After making her morning round with her alms-bowl, she would usually seat herself before a very small loom, to weave cloth much too narrow for serious use. But her webs were bought always by certain shopkeepers who knew her story; and they made her presents of very small cups, tiny flower-vases, and queer dwarf-trees for her garden.

Her greatest pleasure was the companionship of children; and this she never lacked. Japanese child-life, is mostly passed in temple courts; and many happy childhoods were spent in the court of the Amida-ji. All the mothers in that street liked to have their little ones play there, but cautioned them never to laugh at the Bikuni-San. "Sometimes her ways are strange," they would say; "but that is because she once had a little son, who died, and the pain became too great for her mother's heart. So you must be very good and respectful to her."

Good they were, but not quite respectful in the reverential sense. They knew better than to be that. They called her "Bikuni-San" always, and saluted her nicely; but otherwise they treated her like one of themselves. They played games with her; and she gave them tea in extremely small cups, and made for them heaps of rice-cakes not much bigger than peas, and wove upon her loom cloth of cotton and cloth of silk for the robes of their dolls. So she became to them as a blood-sister.

They played with her daily till they grew too big to play, and left the court of the temple of Amida to begin the bitter work of life, and to become the fathers and mothers of children whom they sent to play in their stead. These learned to love the Bikuni-San like their parents had done. And the Bikuni-San lived to play with the children of the children of the children of those who remembered when her temple was built.

The people took good heed that she should not know want. There was always given to her more than she needed for herself. So she was able to be nearly as kind to the children as she wished, and to feed extravagantly certain small animals. Birds nested in her temple, and ate from her hand, and learned not to perch upon the heads of the Buddhas.

Some days after her funeral, a crowd of children visited my house. A little girl of nine years spoke for them all:—

"Sir, we are asking for the sake of the Bikuni-San who is dead. A very large haka(1) has been set up for her. It is a nice haka. But we want to give her also a very, very small haka because in the time she was with us she often said that she would like a very little haka. And the stone-cutter has promised to cut it for us, and to make it very pretty, if we can bring the money. Therefore perhaps you will honorably give something."

"Assuredly," I said. "But now you will have nowhere to play."

She answered, smiling:—"We shall still play in the court of the temple of Amida. She is buried there. She will hear our playing, and be glad."

(1) Tombstone.

VI

AFTER THE WAR

I

Hyogo, May 5, 1895.

Hyogo, this morning, lies bathed in a limpid magnificence of light indescribable,—spring light, which is vapory, and lends a sort of apparitional charm to far things seen through it. Forms remain sharply outlined, but are almost idealized by faint colors not belonging to them; and the great hills behind the town aspire into a cloudless splendor of tint that seems the ghost of azure rather than azure itself.

Over the blue-gray slope of tiled roofs there is a vast quivering and fluttering of extraordinary shapes,—a spectacle not indeed new to me, but always delicious. Everywhere are floating—tied to very tall bamboo poles

—immense brightly colored paper fish, which look and move as if alive. The greater number vary from five to fifteen feet in length; but here and there I see a baby scarcely a foot long, hooked to the tail of a larger one. Some poles have four or five fish attached to them at heights proportioned to the dimensions of the fish, the largest always at the top. So cunningly shaped and colored these things are that the first sight of them is always startling to a stranger. The lines holding them are fastened within the head; and the wind, entering the open mouth, not only inflates the body to perfect form, but keeps it undulating,—rising and descending, turning and twisting, precisely like a real fish, while the tail plays and the fins wave irreproachably. In the garden of my next-door neighbor there are two very fine specimens. One has an orange belly and a bluish-gray back; the other is all a silvery tint; and both have big weird eyes. The rustling of their motion as they swim against the sky is like the sound of wind in a cane-field. A little farther off I see another very big fish, with a little red boy clinging to its back. That red boy represents Kintoki, strongest of all children ever born in Japan, who, while still a baby, wrestled with bears and set traps for goblin-birds.

Everybody knows that these paper carp, or koi, are hoisted only during the period of the great birth festival of boys, in the fifth month; that their presence above a house signifies the birth of a son; and that they symbolize the hope of the parents that their lad will be able to win his way through the world against all obstacles,—even as the real koi, the great Japanese carp, ascends swift rivers against the stream. In many parts of southern and western Japan you rarely see these koi. You see, instead, very long narrow flags of cotton cloth, called nobori, which are fastened perpendicularly, like sails, with little spars and rings to poles of bamboo, and bear designs in various colors of the koi in an eddy,—or of Shoki, conqueror of demons,—or of pines,—or of tortoises,—or other fortunate symbols.

II

But in this radiant spring of the Japanese year 2555, the koi might be taken to symbolize something larger than parental hope, —the great trust of a nation regenerated through war. The military revival of the Empire—the real birthday of New Japan—began with the conquest of China. The war is ended; the future, though clouded, seems big with promise; and, however grim the obstacles to loftier and more enduring achievements, Japan has neither fears nor doubts.

Perhaps the future danger is just in this immense self-confidence. It is not a new feeling created by victory. It is a race feeling, which repeated triumphs have served only to strengthen. From the instant of the declaration of war there was never the least doubt of ultimate victory. There was universal and profound enthusiasm, but no outward signs of emotional excitement. Men at once set to writing histories of the triumphs of Japan, and these histories—issued to subscribers in weekly or monthly parts, and illustrated with photo-lithographs or drawings on wood—were selling all over the country long before any foreign observers could have ventured to predict the final results of the campaign. From first to last the nation felt sure of its own strength, and of the impotence of China. The toy-makers put suddenly into the market legions of ingenious mechanisms, representing Chinese soldiers in flight, or being cut down by Japanese troopers, or tied together as prisoners by their queues, or kowtowing for mercy to illustrious generals. The old-fashioned military playthings, representing samurai in armor, were superseded by figures—in clay, wood, paper, or silk—of Japanese cavalry, infantry, and artillery; by models of forts and batteries; and models of men-of-war. The storming of the defenses of Port Arthur by the Kumamoto Brigade was the subject of one ingenious mechanical toy; another, equally clever, repeated the fight of the Matsushima Kan with the Chinese iron-clads. There were sold likewise myriads of toy-guns discharging corks by compressed air with a loud pop, and myriads of toy-swords, and countless tiny bugles, the constant blowing of which recalled to me the tin-horn tumult of a certain New Year's Eve in New Orleans. The announcement of each victory resulted in an enormous manufacture and sale of colored prints, rudely and cheaply executed, and mostly depicting the fancy of the artist only,—but well fitted to stimulate the popular love of glory. Wonderful sets of chessmen also appeared, each piece representing a Chinese or Japanese officer or soldier.

Meanwhile, the theatres were celebrating the war after a much more complete fashion. It is no exaggeration to say that almost every episode of the campaign was repeated upon the stage. Actors even visited the battlefields to study scenes and backgrounds, and fit themselves to portray realistically, with the aid of artificial snowstorms, the hardships of the army in Manchuria. Every gallant deed was dramatized almost as soon as reported. The death of the bugler Shirakami Genjiro[1]; the triumphant courage of Harada Jiukichi, who scaled a rampart and opened a fortress gate to his comrades; the heroism of the fourteen troopers who held their own against three hundred infantry; the successful charge of unarmed coolies upon a Chinese battalion,—all these and many other incidents were reproduced in a thousand theatres. Immense illuminations of paper lanterns, lettered with phrases of loyalty or patriotic cheer, celebrated the success of the imperial arms, or gladdened the eyes of soldiers going by train to the field. In Kobe,—constantly traversed by troop-trains,—such illuminations continued night after night for weeks together; and the residents of each street further subscribed for flags and triumphal arches.

But the glories of the war were celebrated also in ways more durable by the various great industries of the country. Victories and incidents of sacrificial heroism were commemorated in porcelain, in metal-work, and in costly textures, not less than in new designs for envelopes and note-paper.

They were portrayed on the silk linings of haori(2), on women's kerchiefs of chirimen(3), in the embroidery of girdles, in the designs of silk shirts and of children's holiday robes,—not to speak of cheaper printed goods, such as calicoes and toweling. They were represented in lacquer-ware of many kinds, on the sides and covers of carven boxes, on tobacco-pouches, on sleeve-buttons, in designs for hairpins, on women's combs, even on chopsticks. Bundles of toothpicks in tiny cases were offered for sale, each toothpick having engraved upon it, in microscopic text, a different poem about the war. And up to the time of peace, or at least up to the time of the insane attempt by a soshi(4) to kill the Chinese plenipotentiary during negotiations, all things happened as the people had wished and expected.

But as soon as the terms of peace had been announced, Russia interfered, securing the help of France and Germany to bully Japan. The combination met with no opposition; the government played jiujutsu, and foiled expectations by unlooked-for yielding. Japan had long ceased to feel uneasy about her own military power. Her reserve strength is probably much greater than has ever been acknowledged, and her educational system, with its twenty-six thousand schools, is an enormous drilling-machine. On her own soil she could face any foreign power. Her navy was her weak point, and of this she was fully aware. It was a splendid fleet of small, light cruisers, and splendidly handled. Its admiral, without the loss of a single vessel, had annihilated the Chinese fleet in two engagements, but it was not yet sufficiently heavy to face the combined navies of three European powers; and the flower of the Japanese army was beyond the sea. The most opportune moment for interference had been cunningly chosen, and probably more than interference was intended. The heavy Russian battle-ships were stripped for fighting; and these alone could possibly have overpowered the Japanese fleet, though the victory would have been a costly one. But Russian action was suddenly checked by the sinister declaration of English sympathy for Japan. Within a few weeks England could bring into Asiatic waters a fleet capable of crushing, in one short battle, all the iron-clads assembled by the combination. And a single shot from a Russian cruiser might have plunged the whole world into war.

But in the Japanese navy there was a furious desire to battle with the three hostile powers at once. It would have been a great fight, for no Japanese commander would have dreamed of yielding, no Japanese ship would have struck her colors. The army was equally desirous of war. It needed all the firmness of the government to hold the nation back. Free speech was gagged; the press was severely silenced; and by the return to China of the Liao-Tung peninsula, in exchange for a compensatory increase of the war indemnity previously exacted, peace was secured. The government really acted with faultless wisdom. At this period of Japanese development a costly war with Russia could not fail to have consequences the most disastrous to industry, commerce, and finance. But the national pride has been deeply wounded, and the country can still scarcely forgive its rulers.

(1) At the battle of Song-Hwan, a Japanese bugler named Shirakami Genjiro was ordered to sound the charge (suzume). He had sounded it once when a bullet passed through his lungs, throwing him down.. His comrades tried to take the bugle away, seeing the wound was fatal. He wrested it from them, lifted it again to his lips, sounded the charge once more with all his strength, and fell back dead. I venture to offer this rough translation of a song now sung about him by every soldier and schoolboy in Japan:—

SHIRAKAMI GENJIRO

(After the Japanese military ballad, Rappa-no-hibiki.)
Easy in other times than this
Were Anjo's stream to cross;

But now, beneath the storm of shot,
Its waters seethe and toss.

   In other time to pass that stream
Were sport for boys at play;
But every man through blood must wade
Who fords Anjo to-day.

   The bugle sounds;—through flood and flame
Charges the line of steel;—
Above the crash of battle rings
The bugle's stern appeal.

   Why has that bugle ceased to call?
Why does it call once more?
Why sounds the stirring signal now
More faintly than before?

   What time the bugle ceased to sound,
The breast was smitten through;—
What time the blast rang faintly, blood
Gushed from the lips that blew.

   Death-stricken, still the bugler stands!
He leans upon his gun,—
Once more to sound the bugle-call
Before his life be done.

   What though the shattered body fall?
The spirit rushes free
Through Heaven and Earth to sound anew
That call to Victory!

    Far, far beyond our shore, the spot
Now honored by his fall;—
But forty million brethren
Have heard that bugle-call.

    Comrade!—beyond the peaks and seas
Your bugle sounds to-day
In forty million loyal hearts
A thousand miles away!

(2) Haori, a sort of upper dress, worn by men as well as women. The linings are often of designs beautiful beyond praise.

(3) Chirimen is crape-silk, of which there are many qualities; some very costly and durable.

(4) Soshi form one of the modern curses of Japan. They are mostly ex-students who earn a living by hiring themselves out as rowdy terrorists. Politicians employ them either against the soshi of opponents, or as bullies in election time. Private persons sometimes employ them as defenders. They have figured in most of the election rows which have taken place of late years in Japan, also in a number of assaults made on distinguished personages. The causes which produced nihilism in Russia have several points of resemblance with the causes which developed the modern soshi class in Japan.

III

Hyogo, May 15.

The Matsushima Kan, returned from China, is anchored before the Garden of the Pleasure of Peace. She is not a colossus, though she has done grand things; but she certainly looks quite formidable as she lies there in the clear light,—a stone-gray fortress of steel rising out of the smooth blue. Permission to visit her has been given to the delighted people, who don their best for the occasion, as for a temple festival, and I am suffered to accompany some of them. All the boats in the port would seem to have been hired for the visitors, so huge is the shoal hovering about the ironclad as we arrive. It is not possible for such a number of sightseers to go on board at once, and we have to wait while hundreds are being alternately admitted and dismissed. But the waiting in the cool sea air is not unpleasant; and the spectacle of the popular joy is worth watching. What eager rushing when the turn comes! what swarming and squeezing and clinging! Two women fall into the sea, and are pulled out by blue-jackets, and say they are not sorry to have fallen in, because they can now boast of owing their lives to the men of the Matsushima Kan! As a matter of fact, they could not very well have been drowned; there were legions of common boatmen to look after them.

But something of larger importance to the nation than the lives of two young women is really owing to the men of the Matsushima Kan; and the people are rightly trying to pay them back with love,—for presents, such as thousands would like to make, are prohibited by disciplinary rule. Officers and crew must be weary; but the crowding and the questioning are borne with charming amiability. Everything is shown and explained in detail: the huge thirty-centimetre gun, with its loading apparatus and directing machinery; the quick-firing batteries; the torpedoes, with their impulse-tubes; the electric lantern, with its searching mechanism. I myself, though a foreigner, and therefore requiring a special permit, am guided all about, both below and above, and am even suffered to take a peep at the portraits of their Imperial Majesties, in the admiral's cabin; and I am told the stirring story of the great fight off the Yalu. Meanwhile, the old bald men and the women and the babies of the port hold for one golden day command of the Matsushima. Officers, cadets, blue-jackets, spare no effort to please. Some talk to the grandfathers; others let the children play with the hilts of their swords, or teach them how to throw up their little hands and shout "*Teikoku Banzai!*" And for tired mothers, matting has been spread, where they can squat down in the shade between decks.

Those decks, only a few months ago, were covered with the blood of brave men. Here and there dark stains, which still resist holy-stoning, are visible; and the people look at them with tender reverence. The flagship was twice struck by enormous shells, and her vulnerable parts were pierced by a storm of small projectiles. She bore the brunt of the engagement, losing nearly half her crew. Her tonnage is only four thousand two hundred and eighty; and her immediate antagonists were two Chinese ironclads of seven thousand four hundred tons each. Outside, her cuirass shows no deep scars, for the shattered plates have been replaced;—but my guide points proudly to the numerous patchings of the decks, the steel masting supporting the fighting-tops, the smoke-stack,—and to certain terrible dents, with small cracks radiating from them, in the foot-thick steel of the barbette. He traces for us, below, the course of the thirty-and-a-half centimetre shell that pierced the ship. "When it came," he tells us, "the shock threw men into the air that high" (holding his hand some two feet above the deck). "At the same moment all became dark; you could not see your hand. Then we found that one of the starboard forward guns had been smashed, and the crew all killed. We had forty men killed instantly, and many more wounded: no man escaped in that part of the ship. The deck was on fire, because a lot of ammunition brought up for the guns had exploded; so we had to fight and to work to put out the fire at the same time. Even badly wounded men, with the skin blown from their hands and faces, worked as if they felt no pain; and dying men helped to pass water. But we silenced the Ting-yuen with one more shot from our big gun. The Chinese had European gunners helping them. If we had not had to fight against Western gunners, *our victory would have been too easy.*"

He gives the true note. Nothing, on this splendid spring day, could so delight the men of the Matsushima Kan as a command to clear for action, and attack the great belted Russian cruisers lying off the coast.

IV

Kobe, June 9.

Last year, while traveling from Shimonoseki to the capital, I saw many regiments on their way to the seat of war, all uniformed in white, for the hot season was not yet over. Those soldiers looked so much like students whom I had taught (thousands, indeed, were really fresh from school) that I could not help feeling it was cruel to send such youths to battle. The boyish faces were so frank, so cheerful, so seemingly innocent of the greater sorrows of life! "Don't fear for them," said an English fellow-traveler, a man who had passed his life in camps; "they will give a splendid account of themselves."

"I know it," was my answer; "but I am thinking of fever and frost and Manchurian winter: these are more to be feared than Chinese rifles(1)."

The calling of the bugles, gathering the men together after dark, or signaling the hour of rest, had for years been one of the pleasures of my summer evenings in a Japanese garrison town. But during the months of war, those long, plaintive notes of the last call touched me in another way. I do not know that the melody is peculiar; but it was sometimes played, I used to think, with peculiar feeling; and when uttered to the starlight by all the bugles of a division at once, the multitudinously blending tones had a melancholy sweetness never to be forgotten. And I would dream of phantom buglers, summoning the youth and strength of hosts to the shadowy silence of perpetual rest.

Well, to-day I went to see some of the regiments return. Arches of greenery had been erected over the street they were to pass through, leading from Kobe station to Nanko-San,—the great temple dedicated to the hero spirit of Kusunoki Masashige. The citizens had subscribed six thousand yen for the honor of serving the soldiers with the first meal after their return; and many battalions had already received such kindly welcome. The sheds under which they ate in the court of the temple had been decorated with flags and festoons; and there were gifts for all the troops,—sweetmeats, and packages of cigarettes, and little towels printed with poems in praise of valor. Before the gate of the temple a really handsome triumphal arch had been erected, bearing on each of its facades a phrase of welcome in Chinese text of gold, and on its summit a terrestrial globe surmounted by a hawk with outspread pinions(2).

I waited first, with Manyemon, before the station, which is very near the temple. The train arrived; a military sentry ordered all spectators to quit the platform, and outside, in the street, police kept back the crowd, and stopped all traffic. After a few minutes, the battalions came, marching in regular column through the brick archway,—headed by a gray officer, who limped slightly as he walked, smoking a cigarette. The crowd thickened about us, but there was no cheering, not even speaking,—a hush broken only by the measured tramp of the passing troops. I could scarcely believe those were the same men I had seen going to the war; only the numbers on the shoulder-straps assured me of the fact. Sunburnt and grim the faces were; many had heavy beards. The dark blue winter uniforms were frayed and torn, the shoes worn into shapelessness; but the strong, swinging stride was the stride of the hardened soldier. Lads no longer these, but toughened men, able to face any troops in the world; men who had slaughtered and stormed; men who had also suffered many things which never will be written. The features showed neither joy nor pride; the quick-searching eyes hardly glanced at the welcoming flags, the decorations, the arch with its globe-shadowing hawk of battle, —perhaps because those eyes had seen too often the things which make men serious. (Only one man smiled as he passed; and I thought of a smile seen on the face of a Zouave when I was a boy, watching the return of a regiment from Africa,—a mocking smile, that stabbed.) Many of the spectators were visibly affected, feeling the reason of the change. But, for that, the soldiers were better soldiers now; and they were going to find welcome, and comforts, and gifts, and the great warm love of the people,—and repose thereafter, in their old familiar camps.

I said to Manyemon: "This evening they will be in Osaka and Nagoya. They will hear the bugles calling; and they will think of comrades who never can return."

The old man answered, with simple earnestness: "Perhaps by Western people it is thought that the dead never return. But we cannot so think. There are no Japanese dead who do not return. There are none who do not know the way. From China and from Chosen, and out of the bitter sea, all our dead have come back,—all! They are with us now. In every dusk they gather to hear the bugles that called them home. And they will hear them also in that day when the armies of the Son of Heaven shall be summoned against Russia."

(1) The total number of Japanese actually killed in battle, from the fight at A-san to the capture of the Pescadores, was only 739. But the deaths resulting from other causes, up to as late a date as the 8th of June, during the occupation of Formosa, were 3,148. Of these, 1,602 were due to cholera

alone. Such, at least, were the official figures as published in the Kobe Chronicle.

(2) At the close of the great naval engagement of the 17th of September, 1894, a hawk alighted on the fighting-mast of the Japanese cruiser Takachiho, and suffered itself to be taken and fed. After much petting, this bird of good omen was presented to the Emperor. Falconry was a great feudal sport in Japan, and hawks were finely trained. The hawk is now likely to become, more than ever before in Japan, a symbol of victory.

VII.

HARU

Haru was brought up, chiefly at home, in that old-fashioned way which produced one of the sweetest types of woman the world has ever seen. This domestic education cultivated simplicity of heart, natural grace of manner, obedience, and love of duty as they were never cultivated but in Japan. Its moral product was something too gentle and beautiful for any other than the old Japanese society: it was not the most judicious preparation for the much harsher life of the new,—in which it still survives. The refined girl was trained for the condition of being theoretically at the mercy of her husband. She was taught never to show jealousy, or grief, or anger,—even under circumstances compelling all three; she was expected to conquer the faults of her lord by pure sweetness. In short, she was required to be almost superhuman,—to realize, at least in outward seeming, the ideal of perfect unselfishness. And this she could do with a husband of her own rank, delicate in discernment,—able to divine her feelings, and never to wound them.

Haru came of a much better family than her husband; and she was a little too good for him, because he could not really understand her. They had been married very young, had been poor at first, and then had gradually become well-off, because Haru's husband was a clever man of business. Sometimes she thought he had loved her most when they were less well off; and a woman is seldom mistaken about such matters.

She still made all his clothes; and he commended her needle-work. She waited upon his wants, aided him to dress and undress, made everything comfortable for him in their pretty home; bade him a charming farewell as he went to business in the morning, and welcomed him upon his return; received his friends exquisitely; managed his household matters with wonderful economy, and seldom asked any favors that cost money. Indeed she scarcely needed such favors; for he was never ungenerous, and liked to see her daintily dressed,—looking like some beautiful silver moth robed in the folding of its own wings,—and to take her to theatres and other places of amusement. She accompanied him to pleasure-resorts famed for the blossoming of cherry-trees in spring, or the shimmering of fireflies on summer nights, or the crimsoning of maples in autumn. And sometimes they would pass a day together at Maiko, by the sea, where the pines seem to sway like dancing girls; or an afternoon at Kiyomidzu, in the old, old summer-house, where everything is like a dream of five hundred years ago, —and where there is a great shadowing of high woods, and a song of water leaping cold and clear from caverns, and always the plaint of flutes unseen, blown softly in the antique way,—a tone-caress of peace and sadness blending, just as the gold light glooms into blue over a dying sun.

Except for such small pleasures and excursions, Haru went out seldom. Her only living relatives, and also those of her husband, were far away in other provinces, and she had few visits to make. She liked to be at home, arranging flowers for the alcoves or for the gods, decorating the rooms, and feeding the tame gold-fish of the garden-pond, which would lift up their heads when they saw her coming.

No child had yet brought new joy or sorrow into her life. She looked, in spite of her wife's coiffure, like a very young girl; and she was still simple as a child,—notwithstanding that business capacity in small things which her husband so admired that he often condescended to ask her counsel in big things. Perhaps the heart then judged for him better than the pretty head; but, whether intuitive or not, her advice never proved wrong. She was happy enough with him for five years,—during which time he showed himself as considerate as any young Japanese merchant could well be towards a wife of finer character than his own.

Then his manner suddenly became cold,—so suddenly that she felt assured the reason was not that which a childless wife might have reason to fear. Unable to discover the real cause, she tried to persuade herself that she had been remiss in her duties; examined her innocent conscience to no purpose; and tried very, very hard to please. But he remained unmoved. He spoke no unkind words,— though she felt behind his silence the repressed tendency to utter them. A Japanese of the better class is not very apt to be unkind to his wife in words. It is thought to be vulgar and brutal. The educated man of normal disposition will even answer a wife's reproaches with gentle phrases. Common politeness, by the Japanese code, exacts this attitude from every manly man; moreover, it is the only safe one. A refined and sensitive woman will not long submit to coarse treatment; a spirited one may even kill herself because of something said in a moment of passion, and such a suicide disgraces the husband for the rest of his life. But there are slow cruelties worse than words, and safer,— neglect or indifference, for example, of a sort to arouse jealousy. A Japanese wife has indeed been trained never to show jealousy; but the feeling is older than all training,— old as love, and likely to live as long. Beneath her passionless mask the

Japanese wife feels like her Western sister,—just like that sister who prays and prays, even while delighting some evening assembly of beauty and fashion, for the coming of the hour which will set her free to relieve her pain alone.

Haru had cause for jealousy; but she was too much of a child to guess the cause at once; and her servants too fond of her to suggest it. Her husband had been accustomed to pass his evenings in her company, either at home or elsewhere. But now, evening after evening, he went out by himself. The first time he had given her some business pretexts; afterwards he gave none, and did not even tell her when he expected to return. Latterly, also, he had been treating her with silent rudeness. He had become changed,—"as if there was a goblin in his heart,"—the servants said. As a matter of fact he had been deftly caught in a snare set for him. One whisper from a geisha had numbed his will; one smile blinded his eyes. She was far less pretty than his wife; but she was very skillful in the craft of spinning webs,—webs of sensual delusion which entangle weak men; and always tighten more and more about them until the final hour of mockery and ruin. Haru did not know. She suspected no wrong till after her husband's strange conduct had become habitual,—and even then only because she found that his money was passing into unknown hands. He had never told her where he passed his evenings. And she was afraid to ask, lest he should think her jealous. Instead of exposing her feelings in words, she treated him with such sweetness that a more intelligent husband would have divined all. But, except in business, he was dull. He continued to pass his evenings away; and as his conscience grew feebler, his absences lengthened. Haru had been taught that a good wife should always sit up and wait for her lord's return at night; and by so doing she suffered from nervousness, and from the feverish conditions, that follow sleeplessness, and from the lonesomeness of her waiting after the servants, kindly dismissed at the usual hour, had left her with her thoughts. Once only, returning very late, her husband said to her: "I am sorry you should have sat up so late for me; do not wait like that again!" Then, fearing he might really have been pained on her account, she laughed pleasantly, and said: "I was not sleepy, and I am not tired; honorably please not to think about me." So he ceased to think about her,—glad to take her at her word; and not long after that he stayed away for one whole night. The next night he did likewise, and a third night. After that third night's absence he failed even to return for the morning meal; and Haru knew the time had come when her duty as a wife obliged her to speak.

She waited through all the morning hours, fearing for him, fearing for herself also; conscious at last of the wrong by which a woman's heart can be most deeply wounded. Her faithful servants had told her something; the rest she could guess. She was very ill, and did not know it. She knew only that she was angry— selfishly angry, because of the pain given her, cruel, probing, sickening pain. Midday came as she sat thinking how she could say least selfishly what it was now her duty to say,—the first words of reproach that would ever have passed her lips. Then her heart leaped with a shock that made everything blur and swim before her sight in a whirl of dizziness,—because there was a sound of kuruma-wheels and the voice of a servant calling: "*Honorable-return-is!*"

She struggled to the entrance to meet him, all her slender body a-tremble with fever and pain, and terror of betraying that pain. And the man was startled, because instead of greeting him with the accustomed smile, she caught the bosom of his silk robe in one quivering little hand,—and looked into his face with eyes that seemed to search for some shred of a soul,—and tried to speak, but could utter only the single word, "*Anata(1)?*" Almost in the same moment her weak grasp loosened, her eyes closed with a strange smile; and even before he could put out his arms to support her, she fell. He sought to lift her. But something in the delicate life had snapped. She was dead.

There were astonishments, of course, and tears, and useless callings of her name, and much running for doctors. But she lay white and still and beautiful, all the pain and anger gone out of her face, and smiling as on her bridal day.

Two physicians came from the public hospital,—Japanese military surgeons. They asked straight hard questions,—questions that cut open the self of the man down to the core. Then they told him truth cold and sharp as edged steel,—and left him with his dead.

The people wondered he did not become a priest,—fair evidence that his conscience had been awakened. By day he sits among his bales of Kyoto silks and Osaka figured goods,—earnest and silent. His clerks think him a good master; he never speaks harshly. Often he works far into the night; and he has changed his dwelling-place. There are strangers in the pretty house where Haru lived; and the owner never visits it. Perhaps because he might see there one slender shadow, still arranging flowers, or bending with iris-grace above the goldfish in his pond. But wherever he rest, sometime in the silent hours he must see the same soundless presence near his pillow,—sewing, smoothing, softly seeming to make beautiful the robes he once put on only to betray. And at other times—in the busiest moments of his busy life—the clamor of the great shop dies; the ideographs of his ledger dim and vanish; and a plaintive little voice, which the gods refuse to silence, utters into the solitude of his heart, like a question, the single word,—"*Anata?*" (1) "Thou?"

VIII

A GLIMPSE OP TENDENCIES

I

The foreign concession of an open port offers a striking contrast to its far-Eastern environment. In the well-ordered ugliness of its streets one finds suggestions of places not on this side of the world,—just as though fragments of the Occident had been magically brought oversea: bits of Liverpool, of Marseilles, of New York, of New Orleans, and bits also of tropical towns in colonies twelve or fifteen thousand miles away. The mercantile buildings—immense by comparison with the low light Japanese shops—seem to utter the menace of financial power. The dwellings, of every conceivable design—from that of an Indian bungalow to that of an English or French country-manor, with turrets and bow-windows—are surrounded by commonplace gardens of clipped shrubbery; the white roadways are solid and level as tables, and bordered with boxed-up trees. Nearly all things conventional in England or America have been domiciled in these districts. You see church-steeples and factory-chimneys and telegraph-poles and street-lamps. You see warehouses of imported brick with iron shutters, and shop fronts with plate-glass windows, and sidewalks, and cast-iron railings. There are morning and evening and weekly newspapers; clubs and reading-rooms and bowling alleys; billiard halls and barrooms; schools and bethels. There are electric-light and telephone companies; hospitals, courts, jails, and a foreign police. There are foreign lawyers, doctors, and druggists; foreign grocers, confectioners, bakers, dairymen; foreign dress-makers and tailors; foreign school-teachers and music-teachers. There is a town-hall, for municipal business and public meetings of all kinds,—likewise for amateur theatricals or lectures and concerts; and very rarely some dramatic company, on a tour of the world, halts there awhile to make men laugh and women cry like they used to do at home. There are cricket-grounds, racecourses, public parks,—or, as we should call them in England, "squares,"—yachting associations, athletic societies, and swimming baths. Among the familiar noises are the endless tinkling of piano-practice, the crashing of a town-band, and an occasional wheezing of accordions: in fact, one misses only the organ-grinder. The population is English, French, German, American, Danish, Swedish, Swiss, Russian, with a thin sprinkling of Italians and Levantines. I had almost forgotten the Chinese. They are present in multitude, and have a little corner of the district to themselves. But the dominant element is English and American, the English being in the majority. All the faults and some of the finer qualities of the masterful races can be studied here to better advantage than beyond seas,—because everybody knows all about everybody else in communities so small,—mere oases of Occidental life in the vast unknown of the Far East. Ugly stories may be heard which are not worth writing about; also stories of nobility and generosity—about good brave things done by men who pretend to be selfish, and wear conventional masks to hide what is best in them from public knowledge.

But the domains of the foreigner do not stretch beyond the distance of an easy walk, and may shrink back again into nothing before many years—for reasons I shall presently dwell upon. His settlements developed precociously,—almost like "mushroom cities" in the great American West,—and reached the apparent limit of their development soon after solidifying.

About and beyond the concession, the "native town"—the real Japanese city—stretches away into regions imperfectly known. To the average settler this native town remains a world of mysteries; he may not think it worth his while to enter it for ten years at a time. It has no interest for him, as he is not a student of native customs, but simply a man of business; and he has no time to think how queer it all is. Merely to cross the concession line is almost the same thing as to cross the Pacific Ocean,—which is much less wide than the difference between the races. Enter alone into the interminable narrow maze of Japanese streets, and the dogs will bark at you, and the children stare at you as if you were the only foreigner they ever saw. Perhaps they will even call after you "Ijin," "Tojin," or "Ketojin,"—the last of which signifies "hairy foreigner," and is not intended as a compliment.

II

For a long time the merchants of the concessions had their own way in everything, and forced upon the native firms methods of business to which no Occidental merchant would think of submitting,—methods which plainly expressed the foreign conviction that all Japanese were tricksters. No foreigner would then purchase anything until it had been long enough in his hands to be examined and re-examined and "exhaustively" examined,—or accept any order for imports unless the order were accompanied by "a substantial payment of bargain money"(1). Japanese buyers and sellers protested in vain; they found themselves obliged to submit. But they bided their time,—yielding only with the determination to conquer. The rapid growth of the foreign town, and the immense capital successfully invested therein, proved to them how much they would have to learn before being able to help themselves. They wondered without admiring, and traded with the foreigners or worked for them, while secretly detesting them. In old Japan the merchant ranked below the common peasant; but these foreign invaders assumed the tone of princes and the insolence of conquerors. As employers they were usually harsh, and sometimes brutal. Nevertheless they were wonderfully wise in the matter of making money; they lived like kings and paid high salaries. It was desirable that young men should suffer in their service for the sake of learning things which would have to be learned to save the country from passing under foreign rule. Some day Japan would have a mercantile marine of her own, and foreign banking agencies, and foreign credit, and be well able to rid herself of these haughty strangers: in the meanwhile they should be endured as teachers.

So the import and export trade remained entirely in foreign hands, and it grew from nothing to a value of hundreds of millions; and Japan was well exploited. But she knew that she was only paying to learn; and her patience was of that kind which endures so long as to be mistaken for oblivion of injuries. Her opportunities came in the natural order of things. The growing influx of aliens seeking fortune gave her the first advantage. The intercompetition for Japanese trade broke down old methods; and new firms being glad to take orders and risks without "bargain-money," large advance-payments could no longer be exacted. The relations between foreigners and Japanese simultaneously improved,—as the latter showed a dangerous capacity for sudden combination against ill-treatment, could not be cowed by revolvers, would not suffer abuse of any sort, and knew how to dispose of the most dangerous rowdy in the space of a few minutes. Already the rougher Japanese of the ports, the dregs of the populace, were ready to assume the aggressive on the least provocation.

Within two decades from the founding of the settlements, those foreigners who once imagined it a mere question of time when the whole country would belong to them, began to understand how greatly they had underestimated the race. The Japanese had been learning wonderfully well —"nearly as well as the Chinese." They were supplanting the small foreign shopkeepers; and various establishments had been compelled to close because of Japanese competition. Even for large firms the era of easy fortune-making was over; the period of hard work was commencing. In early days all the personal wants of foreigners had necessarily been supplied by foreigners,—so that a large retail trade had grown up under the patronage of the wholesale trade. The retail trade of the settlements was evidently doomed. Some of its branches had disappeared; the rest were visibly diminishing.

To-day the economic foreign clerk or assistant in a business house cannot well afford to live at the local hotels. He can hire a Japanese cook at a very small sum per month, or can have his meals sent him from a Japanese restaurant at five to seven sen per plate. He lives in a house constructed in "semi-foreign style," and owned by a Japanese. The carpets or mattings on his floor are of Japanese manufacture. His furniture is supplied by a Japanese cabinet-maker. His suits, shirts, shoes, walking-cane, umbrella, are "Japanese make": even the soap on his washstand is stamped with Japanese ideographs. If a smoker, he buys his Manila cigars from a Japanese tobacconist half a dollar cheaper per box than any foreign house would charge him for the same quality. If he wants books he can buy them at much lower prices from a Japanese than from a foreign book dealer,—and select his purchases from a much larger and better-selected stock. If he wants a photograph taken he goes to a Japanese gallery: no foreign photographer could make a living in Japan. If he wants curios he visits a Japanese house; —the foreign dealer would charge him a hundred per cent. dearer.

On the other hand, if he be a man of family, his daily marketing is supplied by Japanese butchers, fishmongers, dairymen, fruit-sellers, vegetable dealers. He may continue for a time to buy English or American hams, bacon, canned goods, etc., from some foreign provision dealer; but he has discovered that Japanese stores now offer the same class of goods at lower prices. If he drinks good beer, it probably comes from a Japanese brewery; and if he wants a good quality of ordinary wine or liquor, Japanese storekeepers can supply it at rates below those of the foreign importer. Indeed, the only things he cannot buy from the Japanese houses are just those things which he cannot afford,—high-priced goods such as only rich men are likely to purchase. And finally, if any of his family become sick, he can consult a Japanese physician who will charge him a fee perhaps one tenth less than he would have had to pay a foreign physician in former times. Foreign doctors now find it very hard to live,—unless they have something more than their practice to rely upon. Even when the foreign doctor brings down his fee to a dollar a visit, the high-class Japanese doctor can charge two, and still crush competition; for, he furnishes the medicine himself at prices which would ruin a foreign apothecary. There are doctors and doctors, of course, as in all countries; but the German-speaking Japanese physician capable of directing a public or military hospital is not easily surpassed in his profession; and the average foreign physician cannot possibly compete with him. He furnishes no prescriptions to be taken to a drugstore: his drugstore is either at home or in a room of the hospital he directs.

These facts, taken at random out of a multitude, imply that foreign shops or as we call them in America, "stores," will soon cease to be. The existence of some has been prolonged only by needless and foolish trickery on the part of some petty Japanese dealers,—attempts to sell abominable decoctions in foreign bottles under foreign labels, to adulterate imported goods, or to imitate trade-marks. But the common sense of the Japanese dealers, as a mass, is strongly opposed to such immorality, and the evil will soon correct itself. The native storekeepers can honestly undersell the foreign ones, because able not only to underlive them, but to make fortunes during the competition.

This has been for some time well recognized in the concessions. But the delusion prevailed that the great exporting and importing firms were impregnable; that they could still control the whole volume of commerce

Really the dullest foreigner could not have believed that a people of forty millions, uniting all their energies to achieve absolute national independence, would remain content to leave the management of their country's import and export trade to aliens, —especially in view of the feeling in the open ports. The existence of foreign settlements in Japan, under consular jurisdiction, was in itself a constant exasperation to national pride,—an indication of national weakness. It had so been proclaimed in print,—in speeches by members of the anti-foreign league,—in speeches made in parliament. But knowledge of the national desire to control the whole of Japanese commerce, and the periodical manifestations of hostility to foreigners as settlers, excited only temporary uneasiness. It was confidently asserted that the Japanese could only injure themselves by any attempt to get rid of foreign negotiators. Though alarmed at the prospect of being brought under Japanese law, the merchants of the concessions never imagined a successful attack upon large interests possible, except by violation of that law itself. It signified little that the Nippon Yusen Kwaisha had become, during the war, one of the largest steamship companies in the world; that Japan was trading directly with India and China; that Japanese banking agencies were being established in the great manufacturing centres abroad; that Japanese merchants were sending their sons to Europe and America for a sound commercial education. Because Japanese lawyers were gaining a large foreign clientele; because Japanese shipbuilders, architects, engineers had replaced foreigners in government service, it did not at all follow that the foreign agents controlling the import and export trade with Europe and America could be dispensed with. The machinery of commerce would be useless in Japanese hands; and capacity for other professions by no means augured latent capacity for business. The foreign capital invested in Japan could not be successfully threatened by any combinations formed against it. Some Japanese houses might carry on a small import business, but the export trade required a thorough knowledge of business conditions on the other side of the world, and such connections and credits as the Japanese could not obtain. Nevertheless the self-confidence of the foreign importers, and exporters was rudely broken in July, 1895, when a British house having brought suit against a Japanese company in a Japanese court, for refusal to accept delivery of goods ordered, and having won a judgment for nearly thirty thousand dollars, suddenly found itself confronted and menaced by a guild whose power had never been suspected. The Japanese firm did not appeal against the decision of the court: it expressed itself ready to pay the whole sum at once—if required. But the guild to which it belonged informed the triumphant plaintiffs that a compromise would be to their advantage. Then the English house discovered itself threatened with a boycott which could utterly ruin it,—a boycott operating in all the industrial centres of the Empire. The compromise was promptly effected at considerable loss to the foreign firm; and the settlements were dismayed. There was much denunciation of the immorality of the proceeding(1). But it was a proceeding against which the law could do nothing; for boycotting cannot be satisfactorily dealt with under law; and it afforded proof positive that the Japanese were able to force foreign firms to submit to their dictation,—by foul means if not by fair. Enormous guilds had been organized by the great industries,—combinations whose moves, perfectly regulated by telegraph, could ruin opposition, and could set at defiance even the judgment of tribunals. The Japanese had attempted boycotting in previous years with so little success that they were deemed incapable of combination. But the new situation showed how well they had learned through defeat, and that with further improvement of organization they could reasonably expect to get the foreign trade under control,—if not into their own hands. It would be the next great step toward the realization of the national desire,—Japan only for the Japanese. Even though the country should be opened to foreign settlement, foreign investments would always be at the mercy of Japanese combinations.

(1) A Kobe merchant of great experience, writing to the Kobe Chronicle of August 7, 1895, observed:—"I am not attempting to defend boycotts; but I firmly believe from what has come to my knowledge that in each and every case there has been provocation irritating the Japanese, rousing their feelings and their sense of justice, and driving them to combination as a defense."

V

The foregoing brief account of existing conditions may suffice to prove the evolution in Japan of a social phenomenon of great significance. Of course the prospective opening of the country under new treaties, the rapid development of its industries, and the vast annual increase in the volume of trade with America and Europe, will probably bring about some increase of foreign settlers; and this temporary result might deceive many as to the inevitable drift of things. But old merchants of experience even now declare that the probable further expansion of the ports will really mean the growth of a native competitive commerce that must eventually dislodge foreign merchants. The foreign settlements, as communities, will disappear: there will remain only some few great agencies, such as exist in all the chief ports of the civilized world; and the abandoned streets of the concessions, and the costly foreign houses on the heights, will be peopled and tenanted by Japanese. Large foreign investments will not be made in the interior. And even Christian mission-work must be left to native missionaries; for just as Buddhism never took definite form in Japan until the teaching of its doctrines was left entirely to Japanese priests,—so Christianity will never take any fixed shape till it has been so remodeled as to harmonize with the emotional and social life of the race. Even thus remodeled it can scarcely hope to exist except in the form of a few small sects.

The social phenomenon exhibited can be best explained by a simile. In many ways a human society may be compared biologically with an individual organism. Foreign elements introduced forcibly into the system of either, and impossible to assimilate, set up irritations and partial disintegration, until eliminated naturally or removed artificially. Japan is strengthening herself through elimination of disturbing elements; and this natural process is symbolized in the resolve to regain possession of all the concessions, to bring about the abolishment of consular jurisdiction, to leave nothing under foreign control within the Empire. It is also manifested in the dismissal of foreign employes, in the resistance offered by Japanese congregations to the authority of foreign missionaries, and in the resolute boycotting of foreign merchants. And behind all this race-movement there is more than race-feeling: there is also the definite conviction that foreign help is proof of national feebleness, and that the Empire remains disgraced before the eyes of the commercial world, so long as its import and export trade are managed by aliens. Several large Japanese firms have quite emancipated themselves from the domination of foreign middlemen; large trade with India and China is being carried on by Japanese steamship companies; and communication with the Southern States of America is soon to be established by the Nippon Yusen Kwaisha, for the direct importation of cotton. But the foreign settlements remain constant sources of irritation; and their commercial conquest by untiring national effort will alone satisfy the country, and will prove, even better than the war with China, Japan's real place among nations. That conquest, I think, will certainly be achieved.

VI

What of the future of Japan? No one can venture any positive prediction on the assumption that existing tendencies will continue far into that future.

Not to dwell upon the grim probabilities of war, or the possibility of such internal disorder as might compel indefinite suspension of the constitution, and lead to a military dictatorship,—a resurrected Shogunate in modern uniform,—great changes there will assuredly be, both for better and for worse. Supposing these changes normal, however, one may venture some qualified predictions, based upon the reasonable supposition that the race will continue, through rapidly alternating periods of action and reaction, to assimilate its new-found knowledge with the best relative consequences.

Physically, I think, the Japanese will become before the close of the next century much superior to what they now are. For such belief there are three good reasons. The first is that the systematic military and gymnastic training of the able-bodied youth of the Empire ought in a few generations to produce results as marked as those of the military system in Germany,—increase in stature, in average girth of chest, in muscular development Another reason is that the Japanese of the cities are taking to a richer diet,—a flesh diet; and that a more nutritive food must have physiological results favoring growth. Immense numbers of little restaurants are everywhere springing up, in which "Western Cooking" is furnished almost as cheaply as Japanese food. Thirdly, the delay of marriage necessitated by education and by military service must result in the production of finer and finer generations of children. As immature marriages become the exception rather than the rule, children of feeble constitution will correspondingly diminish in number. At present the extraordinary differences of stature noticeable in any Japanese crowd seem to prove that the race is capable of great physical development under a severer social discipline.

Moral improvement is hardly to be expected—rather the reverse. The old moral ideals of Japan were at least quite as noble as our own; and men could really live up to them in the quiet benevolent times of patriarchal government. Untruthfulness, dishonesty, and brutal crime were rarer than now, as official statistics show, the percentage of crime having been for some years steadily on the increase—which proves of course, among other things, that the struggle for existence has been intensified. The old standard of chastity, as represented in public opinion, was that of a less developed society than our own; yet I do not believe it can be truthfully asserted that the moral conditions were worse than with us. In one respect they were certainly better; for the virtue of Japanese wives was generally in all ages above suspicion(1). If the morals of men were much more open to reproach, it is not necessary to cite Lecky for evidence as to whether a much better state of things prevails in the Occident. Early marriages were encouraged to guard young men from temptations to irregular life; and it is only fair to suppose that in a majority of cases this result was obtained. Concubinage, the privilege of the rich, had its evil side; but it had also the effect of relieving the wife from the physical strain of rearing many children in rapid succession. The social conditions were so different from those which Western religion assumes to be the best possible, that an impartial judgment of them cannot be ecclesiastical. One fact is indisputable,—that they were unfavorable to professional vice; and in many of the larger fortified towns, —the seats of princes,—no houses of prostitution were suffered to exist. When all things are fairly considered, it will be found that Old Japan might claim, in spite of her patriarchal system, to have been less open to reproach even in the matter of sexual morality than many a Western country. The people were better than their laws asked them to be. And now that the relations of the sexes are to be regulated by new codes,—at a time when new codes are really needed, the changes which it is desirable to bring about cannot result in immediate good. Sudden reforms are not made by legislation. Laws cannot directly create sentiment; and real social progress can be made only through change of ethical feeling developed by long discipline and training. Meanwhile increasing pressure of population and increasing competition must tend, while quickening intelligence, to harden character and develop selfishness.

Intellectually there will doubtless be great progress, but not a progress so rapid as those who think that Japan has really transformed herself in thirty years would have us believe. However widely diffused among the people, scientific education cannot immediately raise the average of practical intelligence to the Western level. The common capacity must remain lower for generations. There will be plenty of remarkable exceptions, indeed; and a new aristocracy of intellect is coming into existence. But the real future of the nation depends rather upon the general capacity of the many than upon the exceptional capacity of the few. Perhaps it depends especially upon the development of the mathematical faculty, which is being everywhere assiduously cultivated. At present this is the weak point; hosts of students being yearly debarred from the more important classes of higher study through inability to pass in mathematics. At the Imperial naval and military colleges, however, such results have been obtained as suffice to show that this weakness will eventually be remedied. The most difficult branches of scientific study, will become less formidable to the children of those who have been able to distinguish themselves in such branches.

In other respects, some temporary retrogression is to be looked for. Just so certainly as Japan has attempted that which is above the normal limit of her powers, so certainly must she fall back to that limit, or, rather, below it. Such retrogression will be natural as well as necessary: it will mean nothing more than a recuperative preparation for stronger and loftier efforts. Signs of it are even now visible in the working of certain state-departments,— notably in that of education. The idea of forcing upon Oriental students a course of study above the average capacity of Western students; the idea of making English the language, or at least one of the languages of the country; and the idea of changing ancestral modes of feeling and thinking for the better by such training, were wild extravagances. Japan must develop her own soul: she cannot borrow another. A dear friend whose life has been devoted to philology once said to me while commenting upon the deterioration of manners among the students of Japan: "*Why, the English language itself has been a demoralizing influence!*" There was much depth in that observation. Setting the whole Japanese nation to study English (the language of a people who are being forever preached to about their "rights," and never about their "duties") was almost an imprudence. The policy was too wholesale as well as too sudden. It involved great waste of money and time, and it helped to sap ethical sentiment. In the future Japan will learn English, just as England learns German. But if this study has been wasted in some directions, it has not been wasted in others. The influence of English has effected modifications in the native tongue, making it richer, more flexible, and more capable of expressing the new forms of thought created by the discoveries of modern science. This influence must long continue. There will be a considerable absorption of English—perhaps also of French and German words—into Japanese: indeed this absorption is already marked in the changing speech of the educated classes, not less than in the colloquial of the ports which is mixed with curious modifications of foreign commercial words. Furthermore, the grammatical structure of Japanese is being influenced; and though I cannot agree with a clergyman who lately declared that the use of the passive voice by Tokyo street-urchins announcing the fall of Port Arthur—("*Ryojunko ga senryo sera-reta!*") represented the working of "divine providence," I do think it afforded some proof that the Japanese language, assimilative like the genius of the race, is showing capacity to meet all demands made upon it by the new conditions.

Perhaps Japan will remember her foreign teachers more kindly in the twentieth century. But she will never feel toward the Occident, as she felt toward China before the Meiji era, the reverential respect due by ancient custom to a beloved instructor; for the wisdom of China was voluntarily sought, while that of the West was thrust upon her by violence. She will have some Christian sects of her own; but she will not remember our American and English missionaries as she remembers even now those great Chinese priests who once educated her youth. And she will not preserve relics of our sojourn, carefully wrapped in septuple coverings of silk, and packed away in dainty whitewood boxes, because we had no new lesson of beauty to teach her,—nothing by which to appeal to her emotions.

(1) The statement has been made that there is no word for chastity in the Japanese language. This is true in the same sense only that we might say there is no word for chastity in the English language,—became such words as honor, virtue, purity, chastity have been adopted into English from other languages. Open any good Japanese-English dictionary and you will find many words for chastity. Just as it would be ridiculous to deny that the word "chastity" is modern English, because it came to us through the French from the Latin, so it is ridiculous to deny that Chinese moral terms, adopted into the Japanese tongue more than a thousand years ago are Japanese to-day. The statement, like a majority of missionary statements on these subjects, is otherwise misleading; for the reader is left to infer the absence of an adjective as well as a noun,—and the purely Japanese adjectives signifying chaste are numerous. The word most commonly used applies to both sexes, —and has the old Japanese sense of firm, strict, resisting, honorable. The deficiency of abstract terms in a language by no means implies the deficiency of concrete moral ideas,—a fact which has been vainly pointed out to missionaries more than once.

BY FORCE OF KARMA

"The face of the beloved and the face of the risen sun cannot be looked at."—Japanese Proverb.

I

Modern science assures us that the passion of first love, so far as the individual may be concerned, is "absolutely antecedent to all relative experience whatever(1)." In other words, that which might well seem to be the most strictly personal of all feelings, is not an individual matter at all. Philosophy discovered the same fact long ago, and never theorized more attractively than when trying to explain the mystery of the passion. Science, so far, has severely limited itself to a few suggestions on the subject. This seems a pity, because the metaphysicians could at no time give properly detailed explanations,—whether teaching that the first sight of the beloved quickens in the soul of the lover some dormant prenatal remembrance of divine truth, or that the illusion is made by spirits unborn seeking incarnation. But science and philosophy both agree as to one all-important fact, that the lovers themselves have no choice, that they are merely the subjects of an influence. Science is even the more positive on this point: it states quite plainly that the dead, not the living, are responsible. There would seem to be some sort of ghostly remembrance in first loves. It is true that science, unlike Buddhism, does not declare that under particular conditions we may begin to recollect our former lives. That psychology which is based upon physiology even denies the possibility of memory-inheritance in this individual sense. But it allows that something more powerful, though more indefinite, is inherited,—the sum of ancestral memories incalculable,—the sum of countless billions of trillions of experiences. Thus can it interpret our most enigmatical sensations,—our conflicting impulses,—our strangest intuitions; all those seemingly irrational attractions or repulsions,—all those vague sadnesses or joys, never to be accounted for by individual experience. But it has not yet found leisure to discourse much to us about first love,—although first love, in its relation to the world invisible, is the very weirdest of all human feelings, and the most mysterious.

In our Occident the riddle runs thus. To the growing youth, whose life is normal and vigorous, there comes a sort of atavistic period in which he begins to feel for the feebler sex that primitive contempt created by mere consciousness of physical superiority. But it is just at the time when the society of girls has grown least interesting to him that he suddenly becomes insane. There crosses his life-path a maiden never seen before,—but little different from other daughters of men,—not at all wonderful to common vision. At the same instant, with a single surging shock, the blood rushes to his heart; and all his senses are bewitched. Thereafter, till the madness ends, his life belongs wholly to that new-found being, of whom he yet knows nothing, except that the sun's light seems more beautiful when it touches her. From that glamour no mortal science can disenthrall him. But whose the witchcraft? Is it any power in the living idol? No, psychology tells us that it is the power of the dead within the idolater. The dead cast the spell. Theirs the shock in the lover's heart; theirs the electric shiver that tingled through his veins at the first touch of one girl's hand.

But why they should want her, rather than any other, is the deeper part of the riddle. The solution offered by the great German pessimist will not harmonize well with scientific psychology. The choice of the dead, evolutionally considered, would be a choice based upon remembrance rather than on prescience. And the enigma is not cheerful.

There is, indeed, the romantic possibility that they want her because there survives in her, as in some composite photograph, the suggestion of each and all who loved them in the past. But there is the possibility also that they want her because there reappears in her something of the multitudinous charm of all the women they loved in vain.

Assuming the more nightmarish theory, we should believe that passion, though buried again and again, can neither die nor rest. They who have vainly loved only seem to die; they really live on in generations of hearts, that their desire may be fulfilled. They wait, perhaps though centuries, for the reincarnation of shapes beloved,—forever weaving into the dreams of youth their vapory composite of memories. Hence the ideals unattainable,—the haunting of troubled souls by the Woman-never-to-be-known.

In the Far East thoughts are otherwise; and what I am about to write concerns the interpretation of the Lord Buddha.

(1) Herbert Spencer, Principles of Psychology: "The Feelings."

II

A priest died recently under very peculiar circumstances. He was the priest of a temple, belonging to one of the older Buddhist sects, in a village near Osaka. (You can see that temple from the Kwan-Setsu Railway, as you go by train to Kyoto.)

He was young, earnest, and extremely handsome—very much too handsome for a priest, the women said. He looked like one of those beautiful figures of Amida made by the great Buddhist statuaries of other days.

The men of his parish thought him a pure and learned priest, in which they were right. The women did not think about his virtue or his learning only: he possessed the unfortunate power to attract them, independently of his own will, as a mere man. He was admired by them, and even by women of other parishes also, in ways not holy; and their admiration interfered with his studies and disturbed his meditations. They found irreproachable pretexts for visiting the temple at all hours, just to look at him and talk to him; asking questions which it was his duty to answer, and making religious offerings which he could not well refuse. Some would ask questions, not of a religious kind, that caused him to blush. He was by nature too gentle to protect himself by severe speech, even when forward girls from the city said things that country-girls never would have said,—things that made him tell the speakers to leave his presence. And the more he shrank from the admiration of the timid, or the adulation of the unabashed, the more the persecution increased, till it became the torment of his life(1).

His parents had long been dead; he had no worldly ties: he loved only his calling, and the studies belonging to it; and he did not wish to think of foolish and forbidden things. His extraordinary beauty—the beauty of a living idol—was only a misfortune. Wealth was offered him under conditions that he could not even discuss. Girls threw themselves at his feet, and prayed him in vain to love them. Love-letters were constantly being sent to him, letters which never brought a reply. Some were written in that classical enigmatic style which speaks of "the Rock-Pillow of Meeting," and "waves on the shadow of a face," and "streams that part to reunite." Others were artless and frankly tender, full of the pathos of a girl's first confession of love.

For a long time such letters left the young priest as unmoved, to outward appearance, as any image of that Buddha in whose likeness he seemed to have been made. But, as a matter of fact, he was not a Buddha, but only a weak man; and his position was trying.

One evening there came to the temple a little boy who gave him a letter, whispered the name of the sender, and ran away in the dark. According to the subsequent testimony of an acolyte, the priest read the letter, restored it to its envelope, and placed it on the matting, beside his kneeling cushion. After remaining motionless for a long time, as if buried in thought, he sought his writing-box, wrote a letter himself, addressed it to his spiritual superior, and left it upon the writing-stand. Then he consulted the clock, and a railway time-table in Japanese. The hour was early; the night windy and dark. He prostrated himself for a moment in prayer before the altar; then hurried out into the blackness, and reached the railway exactly in time to kneel down in the middle of the track, facing the roar and rush of the express from Kobe. And, in another moment, those who had worshiped the strange beauty of the man would have shrieked to see, even by lantern-light, all that remained of his poor earthliness, smearing the iron way.

The letter written to his superior was found. It contained a bare statement to the effect that, feeling his spiritual strength departing from him, he had resolved to die in order that he might not sin.

The other letter was still lying where he had left it on the floor,—a letter written in that woman-language of which every syllable is a little caress of humility. Like all such letters (they are never sent through the post) it contained no date, no name, no initial, and its envelope bore no address. Into our incomparably harsher English speech it might be imperfectly rendered as follows:—

To take such freedom may be to assume overmuch; yet I feel that I must speak to you, and therefore send this letter. As for my lowly self, I have to say only that when first seeing you in the period of the Festival of the Further Shore, I began to think; and that since then I have not, even for a moment, been able to forget. More and more each day I sink into that ever-growing thought of you; and when I sleep I dream; and when, awaking and seeing you not, I remember there was no truth in my thoughts of the night, I can do nothing but weep. Forgive me that, having been born into this world a woman, I should utter my wish for the exceeding favor of being found not hateful to one so high. Foolish and without delicacy I may seem in allowing my heart to be thus tortured by the thought of one so far above me. But only because knowing that I cannot restrain my heart, out of the depth of it I have suffered these poor words to come, that I may write them with my unskillful brush, and send them to you. I pray that you will deem me worthy of pity; I beseech that you will not send me cruel words in return. Compassionate me, seeing that this is but the overflowing of my humble feelings; deign to divine and justly to judge,—be it only with the least of kindliness,—this heart that, in its great distress alone, so ventures to address you. Each moment I shall hope and wait for some gladdening answer.

Concerning all things fortunate, felicitation.

To-day,— from the honorably-known, to the longed-for, beloved, august one, this letter goes.

(1) Actors in Japan often exercise a similar fascination upon sensitive girls of the lower classes, and often take cruel advantage of the power so gained. It is very rarely, indeed, that such fascination can be exerted by a priest.

III

I called upon a Japanese friend, a Buddhist scholar, to ask some questions about the religious aspects of the incident. Even as a confession of human weakness, that suicide appeared to me a heroism.

It did not so appear to my friend. He spoke words of rebuke. He reminded me that one who even suggested suicide as a means of escape from sin had been pronounced by the Buddha a spiritual outcast,—unfit to live with holy men. As for the dead priest, he had been one of those whom the Teacher called fools. Only a fool could imagine that by destroying his own body he was destroying also within himself the sources of sin.

"But," I protested, "this man's life was pure…. Suppose he sought death that he might not, unwittingly, cause others to commit sin?"

My friend smiled ironically. Then he said:—"There was once a lady of Japan, nobly torn and very beautiful, who wanted to become a nun. She went to a certain temple, and made her wish known. But the high-priest said to her, 'You are still very young. You have lived the life of courts. To the eyes of worldly men you are beautiful; and, because of your face, temptations to return to the pleasures of the world will be devised for you. Also this wish of yours may be due to some momentary sorrow. Therefore, I cannot now consent to your request.' But she still pleaded so earnestly, that he deemed it best to leave her abruptly. There was a large hibachi—a brazier of glowing charcoal—in the room where she found herself alone. She heated the iron tongs of the brazier till they were red, and with them horribly pierced and seamed her face, destroying her beauty forever. Then the priest, alarmed by the smell of the burning, returned in haste, and was very much grieved by what he saw. But she pleaded again, without any trembling in her voice: 'Because I was beautiful, you refused to take me. Will you take me now?' She was accepted into the Order, and became a holy nun…. Well, which was the wiser, that woman, or the priest you wanted to praise?"

"But was it the duty of the priest," I asked, "to disfigure his face?"

"Certainly not! Even the woman's action would have been very unworthy if done only as a protection against temptation. Self-mutilation of any sort is forbidden by the law of Buddha; and she transgressed. But, as she burned her face only that she might be able to enter at once upon the Path, and not because afraid of being unable by her own will to resist sin, her fault was a minor fault. On the other hand, the priest who took his own life committed a very great offense. He should have tried to convert those who tempted him. This he was too weak to do. If he felt it impossible to keep from sinning as a priest, then it would have been better for him to return to the world, and there try to follow the law for such as do not belong to the Order."

"According to Buddhism, therefore, he has obtained no merit?" I queried.

"It is not easy to imagine that he has. Only by those ignorant of the Law can his action be commended."

"And by those knowing the Law, what will be thought of the results, the karma of his act?"

My friend mused a little; then he said, thoughtfully:—"The whole truth of that suicide we cannot fully know. Perhaps it was not the first time."

"Do you mean that in some former life also he may have tried to escape from sin by destroying his own body?"

"Yes. Or in many former lives."

"What of his future lives?"

"Only a Buddha could answer that with certain knowledge."

"But what is the teaching?"

"You forget that it is not possible for us to know what was in the mind of that man."

"Suppose that he sought death only to escape from sinning?"

"Then he will have to face the like temptation again and again, and all the sorrow of it, and all the pain, even for a thousand times a thousand times, until he shall have learned to master himself. There is no escape through death from the supreme necessity of self-conquest."

After parting with my friend, his words continued to haunt me; and they haunt me still. They forced new thoughts about some theories hazarded in the first part of this paper. I have not yet been able to assure myself that his weird interpretation of the amatory mystery is any less worthy of consideration than our Western interpretations. I have been wondering whether the loves that lead to death might not mean much more than the ghostly hunger of buried passions. Might they not signify also the inevitable penalty of long-forgotten sins?

X

A CONSERVATIVE

Amazakaru
Hi no iru kuni ni
Kite wa aredo,
Yamato-nishiki no
Iro wa kawaraji.

I

He was born in a city of the interior, the seat of a daimyo of three hundred thousand koku, where no foreigner had ever been. The yashiki of his father, a samurai of high rank, stood within the outer fortifications surrounding the prince's castle. It was a spacious yashiki; and behind it and around it were landscape gardens, one of which contained a small shrine of the god of armies. Forty years ago there were many such homes. To artist eyes the few still remaining seem like fairy palaces, and their gardens like dreams of the Buddhist paradise.

But sons of samurai were severely disciplined in those days; and the one of whom I write had little time for dreaming. The period of caresses was made painfully brief for him. Even before he was invested with his first hakama, or trousers,—a great ceremony in that epoch,—he was weaned as far as possible from tender influence, and taught to check the natural impulses of childish affection. Little comrades would ask him mockingly, "Do you still need milk?" if they saw him walking out with his mother, although he might love her in the house as demonstratively as he pleased, during the hours he could pass by her side. These were not many. All inactive pleasures were severely restricted by his discipline; and even comforts, except during illness, were not allowed him. Almost from the time he could speak he was enjoined to consider duty the guiding motive of life, self-control the first requisite of conduct, pain and death matters of no consequence in the selfish sense.

There was a grimmer side to this Spartan discipline, designed to cultivate a cold sternness never to be relaxed during youth, except in the screened intimacy of the home. The boys were inured to sights of blood. They were taken to witness executions; they were expected to display no emotion; and they were obliged, on their return home, to quell any secret feeling of horror by eating plentifully of rice tinted blood-color by an admixture of salted plum juice. Even more difficult things might be demanded of a very young boy,—to go alone at midnight to the execution-ground, for example, and bring back a head in proof of courage. For the fear of the dead was held not less contemptible in a samurai than the fear of man. The samurai child was pledged to fear nothing. In all such tests, the demeanor exacted was perfect impassiveness; any swaggering would have been judged quite as harshly as any sign of cowardice.

As a boy grew up, he was obliged to find his pleasures chiefly in those bodily exercises which were the samurai's early and constant preparations for war,—archery and riding, wrestling and fencing. Playmates were found for him; but these were older youths, sons of retainers, chosen for ability to assist him in the practice of martial exercises. It was their duty also to teach him how to swim, to handle a boat, to develop his young muscles. Between such physical training and the study of the Chinese classics the greater part of each day was divided for him. His diet, though ample, was never dainty; his clothing, except in time of great ceremony, was light and coarse; and he was not allowed the use of fire merely to warm himself. While studying of winter mornings, if his hands became too cold to use the writing brush, he would be ordered to plunge them into icy water to restore the circulation; and if his feet were numbed by frost, he would be told to run about in the snow to make them warm. Still more rigid was his training in the special etiquette of the military class, and he was early made to know that the little sword in his girdle was neither an ornament nor a plaything. He was shown how to use it, how to take his own life at a moment's notice, without shrinking, whenever the code of his class might so order(1).

Also in the matter of religion, the training of a samurai boy was peculiar. He was educated to revere the ancient gods and the spirits of his ancestors; he was well schooled in the Chinese ethics; and he was taught something of

Buddhist philosophy and faith. But he was likewise taught that hope of heaven and fear of hell were for the ignorant only; and that the superior man should be influenced in his conduct by nothing more selfish than the love of right for its own sake, and the recognition of duty as a universal law.

Gradually, as the period of boyhood ripened into youth, his conduct was less subjected to supervision. He was left more and more free to act upon his own judgment,—but with full knowledge that a mistake would not be forgotten; that a serious offense would never be fully condoned, and that a well-merited reprimand was more to be dreaded than death. On the other hand, there were few moral dangers against which to guard him. Professional vice was then strictly banished from many of the provincial castle-towns; and even so much of the non-moral side of life as might have been reflected in popular romance and drama, a young samurai could know little about. He was taught to despise that common literature appealing either to the softer emotions or the passions, as essentially unmanly reading; and the public theatre was forbidden to his class(2). Thus, in that innocent provincial life of Old Japan, a young samurai might grow up exceptionally pure-minded and simple-hearted.

So grew up the young samurai concerning whom these things are written, —fearless, courteous, self-denying, despising pleasure, and ready at an instant's notice to give his life for love, loyalty, or honor. But though already a warrior in frame and spirit, he was in years scarcely more than a boy when the country was first startled by the coming of the Black Ships.

II

The policy of Iyemitsu, forbidding any Japanese to leave the country under pain of death, had left the nation for two hundred years ignorant of the outer world. About the colossal forces gathering beyond seas nothing was known. The long existence of the Dutch settlement at Nagasaki had in no wise enlightened Japan as to her true position,—an Oriental feudalism of the sixteenth century menaced by a Western world three centuries older. Accounts of the real wonders of that world would have sounded to Japanese ears like stories invented to please children, or have been classed with ancient tales of the fabled palaces of Horai. The advent of the American fleet, "the Black Ships," as they were then called, first awakened the government to some knowledge of its own weakness, and of danger from afar.

National excitement at the news of the second coming of the Black Ships was followed by consternation at the discovery that the Shogunate confessed its inability to cope with the foreign powers. This could mean only a peril greater than that of the Tartar invasion in the days of Hojo Tokimune, when the people had prayed to the gods for help, and the Emperor himself, at Ise, had besought the spirits of his fathers. Those prayers had been answered by sudden darkness, a sea of thunder, and the coming of that mighty wind still called Kami-kaze,—"the Wind of the Gods," by which the fleets of Kublai Khan were given to the abyss. Why should not prayers now also be made? They were, in countless homes and at thousands of shrines. But the Superior Ones gave this time no answer; the Kami-kaze did not come. And the samurai boy, praying vainly before the little shrine of Hachiman in his father's garden, wondered if the gods had lost their power, or if the people of the Black Ships were under the protection of stronger gods.

(1) "Is that really the head of your father?" a prince once asked of a samurai boy only seven years old. The child at once realized the situation. The freshly-severed head set before him was not his father's: the daimyo had been deceived, but further deception was necessary. So the lad, after

having saluted the head with every sign of reverential grief, suddenly cut out his own bowels. All the prince's doubts vanished before that bloody proof of filial piety; the outlawed father was able to make good his escape, and the memory of the child is still honored in Japanese drama and poetry.

(2) Samurai women, in some province, at least, could go to the public theatre. The men could not,—without committing a breach of good manners. But in samurai homes, or within the grounds of the yashiki, some private performances of a particular character were given. Strolling players were the performers. I know several charming old samurai who have never been to a public theatre in their lives, and refuse all invitations to witness a performance. They still obey the rules of their samurai education.

III

It soon became evident that the foreign "barbarians" were not to be driven away. Hundreds had come, from the East as well as from the West; and all possible measures for their protection had been taken; and they had built queer cities of their own upon Japanese soil. The government had even commanded that Western knowledge was to be taught in all schools; that the study of English was to be made an important branch of public education; and that public education itself was to be remodeled upon Occidental lines. The government had also declared that the future of the country would depend upon the study and mastery of the languages and the science of the foreigners. During the interval, then, between such study and its successful results, Japan would practically remain under alien domination. The fact was not, indeed, publicly stated in so many words; but the signification of the policy was unmistakable. After the first violent emotions provoked by knowledge of the situation,—after the great dismay of the people, and the suppressed fury of the samurai,—there arose an intense curiosity regarding the appearance and character of those insolent strangers who had been able to obtain what they wanted by mere display of superior force. This general curiosity was partly satisfied by an immense production and distribution of cheap colored prints, picturing the manner and customs of the barbarians, and the extraordinary streets of their settlements. Caricatures only those flaring wood—prints could have seemed to foreign eyes. But caricature was not the conscious object of the artist. He tried to portray foreigners as he really saw them; and he saw them as green-eyed monsters, with red hair like Shojo(1), and with noses like Tengu(2), wearing clothes of absurd forms and colors; and dwelling in structures like storehouses or prisons. Sold by hundreds of thousands throughout the interior, these prints must have created many uncanny ideas. Yet as attempts to depict the unfamiliar they were only innocent. One should be able to study those old drawings in order to comprehend just how we appeared to the Japanese of that era; how ugly, how grotesque, how ridiculous.

The young samurai of the town soon had the experience of seeing a real Western foreigner, a teacher hired for them by the prince. He was an Englishman. He came under the protection of an armed escort; and orders were given to treat him as a person of distinction. He did not seem quite so ugly as the foreigners in the Japanese prints: his hair was red, indeed, and his eyes of a strange color; but his face was not disagreeable. He at once became, and long remained, the subject of tireless observation. How closely his every act was watched could never be guessed by any one ignorant of the queer superstitions of the pre-Meiji era concerning ourselves. Although recognized as intelligent and formidable creatures, Occidentals were not generally regarded as quite human; they were thought of as more closely allied to animals than to mankind. They had hairy bodies of queer shape; their teeth were different from those of men; their internal organs were also peculiar; and their moral ideas those of goblins. The timidity which foreigners then inspired, not, indeed, to the samurai, but to the common people, was not a physical, but a superstitious fear. Even the Japanese peasant has never been a coward. But to know his feelings in that time toward foreigners, one must also know something of the ancient beliefs, common to both Japan and China, about animals gifted with supernatural powers, and capable of assuming human form; about the existence of races half-human and half-superhuman; and about the mythical beings of the old picture-books,—goblins long-legged and long-armed and bearded (ashinaga and tenaga), whether depicted by the illustrators of weird stories or comically treated by the brush of Hokusai. Really the aspect of the new strangers seemed to afford confirmation of the fables related by a certain Chinese Herodotus; and the clothing they wore might seem to have been devised for the purpose of hiding what would prove them not human. So the new English teacher, blissfully ignorant of the fact, was studied surreptitiously, just as one might study a curious animal! Nevertheless, from his students he experienced only courtesy: they treated him by that Chinese code which ordains that "even the shadow of a teacher must not be trodden on." In any event it would have mattered little to samurai students whether their teacher were perfectly human or not, so long as he could teach. The hero Yoshitsune had been taught the art of the sword by a Tengu. Beings not human had proved themselves scholars and poets(3). But behind the never-lifted mask of delicate courtesy, the stranger's habits were minutely noted; and the ultimate judgment, based upon the comparison of such observation, was not altogether flattering. The teacher himself could never have imagined the comments made upon him by his two-sworded pupils; nor would it have increased his peace of mind, while overlooking compositions in the class-room, to have understood their conversation:—

"See the color of his flesh, how soft it is! To take off his head with a single blow would be very easy."

Once he was induced to try their mode of wrestling, just for fun, he supposed. But they really wanted to take his physical measure. He was not very highly estimated as an athlete.

"Strong arms he certainly has," one said. "But he does not know how to use his body while using his arms; and his loins are very weak. To break his back would not be difficult."

"I think," said another, "that it would be easy to fight with foreigners."

"With swords it would be very easy," responded a third; "but they are more skilful than we in the use of guns and cannon."

"We can learn all that," said the first speaker. "When we have learned Western military matters, we need not care for Western soldiers."

"Foreigners," observed another, "are not hardy like we are. They soon tire, and they fear cold. All winter our teacher must have a great fire in his room. To stay there five minutes gives me the headache."

But for all that, the lads were kind to their teacher, and made him love them.

(1) Apish mythological beings with red hair, delighting in drunkenness.

(2) Mythological beings of several kinds, supposed to live in the mountains. Some have long noses.

(3) There is a legend that when Toryoko, a great poet, who was the teacher of Sugiwara-no-Michizane (now deified as Tenjin), was once passing the Gate called Ra-jo-mon, of the Emperor's palace at Kyoto, he recited aloud this single verse which he had just composed:—

"Clear is the weather and fair;—and the wind waves the hair of young willows."

Immediately a deep mocking voice from the gateway continued the poem, thus:—

"Melted and vanished the ice; the waves comb the locks of old mosses."

Toryoko looked, but there was no one to be seen. Reaching home, he told his pupil about the matter, and repeated the two compositions. Sugiwara-no-Michizane praised the second one, saying:—

"Truly the words of the first are the words of a poet; but the words of the second are the words of a Demon!"

IV

Changes came as great earthquakes come, without warning: the transformation of daimyates into prefectures, the suppression of the military class, the reconstruction of the whole social system. These events filled the youth with sadness, although he felt no difficulty in transferring his allegiance from prince to emperor, and although the wealth of his family remained unimpaired by the shock. All this reconstruction told him of the greatness of the national danger, and announced the certain disappearance of the old high ideals, and of nearly all things loved. But he knew regret was vain. By self-transformation alone could the nation hope to save its independence; and the obvious duty of the patriot was to recognize necessity, and fitly prepare himself to play the man in the drama of the future.

In the samurai school he had learned much English, and he knew himself able to converse with Englishmen. He cut his long hair, put away his swords, and went to Yokohama that he might continue his study of the language under more favorable conditions. At Yokohama everything at first seemed to him both unfamiliar and repellent. Even the Japanese of the port had been changed by foreign contact: they were rude and rough; they acted and spoke as common people would not have dared to do in his native town. The foreigners themselves impressed him still more disagreeably: it was the period when new settlers could assume the tone of conquerors to the conquered, and when the life of the "open ports" was much less decorous than now. The new buildings of brick or stuccoed timber revived for him unpleasant memories of the Japanese colored pictures of foreign manners and customs; and he could not quickly banish the fancies of his boyhood concerning Occidentals. Reason, based on larger knowledge and experience, fully assured him what they really were; but to his emotional life the intimate sense of their kindred humanity still failed to come. Race-feeling is older than intellectual development; and the superstitions attaching to race-feeling are not easy to get rid of. His soldier-spirit, too, was stirred at times by ugly things heard or seen,—incidents that filled him with the hot impulse of his fathers to avenge a cowardice or to redress a wrong. But he learned to conquer his repulsions as obstacles to knowledge: it was the patriot's duty to study calmly the nature of his country's foes. He trained himself at last to observe the new life about him without prejudice, —its merits not less than its defects; its strength not less than its weakness. He found kindness; he found devotion to ideals,—ideals not his own, but which he knew how to respect because they exacted, like the religion of his ancestors, abnegation of many things.

Through such appreciation he learned to like and to trust an aged missionary entirely absorbed in the work of educating and proselytizing. The old man was especially anxious to convert this young samurai, in whom aptitudes of no common order were discernible; and he spared no pains to win the boy's confidence. He aided him in many ways, taught him something of French and German, of Greek and Latin, and placed entirely at his disposal a private library of considerable extent. The use of a foreign library, including works of history, philosophy, travel, and fiction, was not a privilege then easy for Japanese students to obtain. It was gratefully appreciated; and the owner of the library found no difficulty at a later day in persuading his favored and favorite pupil to read a part of the New Testament. The youth expressed surprise at finding among the doctrines of the "Evil Sect" ethical precepts like those of Confucius. To the old missionary he said: "This teaching is not new to us; but it is certainly very good. I shall study the book and think about it."

V

The study and the thinking were to lead the young man much further than he had thought possible. After the recognition of Christianity as a great religion came recognitions of another order, and various imaginings about the civilization of the races professing Christianity. It then seemed to many reflective Japanese, possibly even to the keen minds directing the national policy, that Japan was doomed to pass altogether under alien rule. There was hope, indeed; and while even the ghost of hope remained, the duty for all was plain. But the power that could be used against the Empire was irresistible. And studying the enormity of that power, the young Oriental could not but ask himself, with a wonder approaching awe, whence and how it had been gained. Could it, as his aged teacher averred, have some occult relation to a higher religion? Certainly the ancient Chinese philosophy, which declared the prosperity of peoples proportionate to their observance of celestial law and their obedience to the teaching of sages, countenanced such a theory. And if the superior force of Western civilization really indicated the superior character of Western ethics, was it not the plain duty of every patriot to follow that higher faith, and to strive for the conversion of the whole nation? A youth of that era, educated in Chinese wisdom, and necessarily ignorant of the history of social evolution in the West, could never have imagined that the very highest forms of material progress were developed chiefly through a merciless competition out of all harmony with Christian idealism, and at variance with every great system of ethics. Even to-day in the West unthinking millions imagine some divine connection between military power and Christian belief, and utterances are made in our pulpits implying divine justification for political robberies, and heavenly inspiration for the invention of high explosives. There still survives among us the superstition that races professing Christianity are divinely destined to rob or exterminate races holding other beliefs. Some men occasionally express their conviction that we still worship Thor and Odin,—the only difference being that Odin has become a mathematician, and that the Hammer Mjolnir is now worked by steam. But such persons are declared by the missionaries to be atheists and men of shameless lives.

Be this as it may, a time came when the young samurai resolved to proclaim himself a Christian, despite the opposition of his kindred. It was a bold step; but his early training had given him firmness; and he was not to be moved from his decision even by the sorrow of his parents. His rejection of the ancestral faith would signify more than temporary pain for him: it would mean disinheritance, the contempt of old comrades, loss of rank, and all the consequences of bitter poverty. But his samurai training had taught him to despise self. He saw what he believed to be his duty as a patriot and as a truthseeker, and he followed it without fear or regret.

VI

Those who hope to substitute their own Western creed in the room of one which they wreck by the aid of knowledge borrowed from modern science, do not imagine that the arguments used against the ancient faith can be used with equal force against the new. Unable himself to reach the higher levels of modern thought, the average missionary cannot foresee the result of his small teaching of science upon an Oriental mind naturally more powerful than his own. He is therefore astonished and shocked to discover that the more intelligent his pupil, the briefer the term of that pupil's Christianity. To destroy personal faith in a fine mind previously satisfied with Buddhist cosmogony, because innocent of science, is not extremely difficult. But to substitute, in the same mind, Western religious emotions for Oriental, Presbyterian or Baptist dogmatisms for Chinese and Buddhist ethics, is not possible. The psychological difficulties in the way are never recognized by our modern evangelists. In former ages, when the faith of the Jesuits and the friars was not less superstitious than the faith they strove to supplant, the same deep-lying obstacles existed; and the Spanish priest, even while accomplishing marvels by his immense sincerity and fiery zeal, must have felt that to fully realize his dream he would need the sword of the Spanish soldier. To-day the conditions are far less favorable for any work of conversion than they ever were in the sixteenth century. Education has been secularized and remodeled upon a scientific basis; our religions are being changed into mere social recognitions of ethical necessities; the functions of our clergy are being gradually transformed into those of a moral police; and the multitude of our church-spires proves no increase of our faith, but only the larger growth of our respect for conventions. Never can the conventions of the Occident become those of the Far East; and never will foreign missionaries be suffered in Japan to take the role of a police of morals. Already the most liberal of our churches, those of broadest culture, begin to recognize the vanity of missions. But it is not necessary to drop old dogmatisms in order to perceive the truth: thorough education should be enough to reveal it; and the most educated of nations, Germany, sends no missionaries to work in the interior of Japan. A result of missionary efforts, much more significant than the indispensable yearly report of new conversions, has been the reorganization of the native religions, and a recent government mandate insisting upon the higher education of the native priest-hoods. Indeed, long before this mandate the wealthier sects had established Buddhist schools on the Western plan; and the Shinshu could already boast of its scholars, educated in Paris or at Oxford,—men whose names are known to Sanscritists the world over. Certainly Japan will need higher forms of faith than her mediaeval ones; but these must be themselves evolved from the ancient forms,—from within, never from without. A Buddhism strongly fortified by Western science will meet the future needs of the race.

The young convert at Yokohama proved a noteworthy example of missionary failures. Within a few years after having sacrificed a fortune in order to become a Christian,—or rather the member of a foreign religious sect,—he publicly renounced the creed accepted at such a cost. He had studied and comprehended the great minds of the age better than his religious teachers, who could no longer respond to the questions he propounded, except by the assurance that books of which they had recommended him to study parts were dangerous to faith as wholes. But as they could not prove the fallacies alleged to exist in such books, their warnings availed nothing. He had been converted to dogmatism by imperfect reasoning; by larger and deeper reasoning he found his way beyond dogmatism. He passed from the church after an open declaration that its tenets were not based upon true reason or fact; and that he felt himself obliged to accept the opinions of men whom his teachers had called the enemies of Christianity. There was great scandal at his "relapse."

The real "relapse" was yet far away. Unlike many with a similar experience, he knew that the religious question had only receded for him, and that all he had learned was scarcely more than the alphabet of what remained to learn. He had not lost belief in the relative value of creeds,—in the worth of religion as a conserving and restraining force. A distorted perception of one truth—the truth of a relation subsisting between civilizations and their religions—had first deluded him into the path that led to his conversion. Chinese philosophy had taught him that which modern sociology recognizes in the law that societies without priesthoods have never developed; and Buddhism had taught him that even delusions—the parables, forms, and symbols presented as actualities to humble minds—have their value and their justification in aiding the development of human goodness. From such a point of view, Christianity had lost none of its interest for him; and though doubting what his teacher had told him about the superior morality of Christian nations, not at all illustrated in the life of the open ports, he desired to see for himself the influence of religion upon morals in the Occident; to visit European countries and to study the causes of their development and the reason of their power.

This he set out to do sooner than he had purposed. That intellectual quickening which had made him a doubter in religious matters had made him also a freethinker in politics. He brought down upon himself the wrath of the government by public expressions of opinion antagonistic to the policy of the hour; and, like others equally imprudent under the stimulus of new ideas, he was obliged to leave the country. Thus began for him a series of wanderings destined to carry him round the world. Korea first afforded him a refuge; then China, where he lived as a teacher; and at last he found himself on board a steamer bound for Marseilles. He had little money; but he did not ask himself how he was going to live in Europe. Young, tall, athletic, frugal and inured to hardship, he felt sure of himself; and he had letters to men abroad who could smooth his way.

But long years were to pass before he could see his native land again.

VII

During those years he saw Western civilization as few Japanese ever saw it; for he wandered through Europe and America, living in many cities, and toiling in many capacities,—sometimes with his brain, oftener with his hands,—and so was able to study the highest and the lowest, the best and the worst of the life about him. But he saw with the eyes of the Far East; and the ways of his judgments were not as our ways. For even as the Occident regards the Far East, so does the Far East regard the Occident, — only with this difference: that what each most esteems in itself is least likely to be esteemed by the other. And both are partly right and partly wrong; and there never has been, and never can be, perfect mutual comprehension.

Larger than all anticipation the West appeared to him,—a world of giants; and that which depresses even the boldest Occidental who finds himself, without means or friends, alone in a great city, must often have depressed the Oriental exile: that vague uneasiness aroused by the sense of being invisible to hurrying millions; by the ceaseless roar of traffic drowning voices; by monstrosities of architecture without a soul; by the dynamic display of wealth forcing mind and hand, as mere cheap machinery, to the uttermost limits of the possible. Perhaps he saw such cities as Dore saw London: sullen majesty of arched glooms and granite deeps opening into granite deeps beyond range of vision, and mountains of masonry with seas of labor in turmoil at their base, and monumental spaces displaying the grimness of ordered power slow-gathering through centuries. Of beauty there was nothing to make appeal to him between those endless cliffs of stone which walled out the sunrise and the sunset, the sky and the wind. All that which draws us to great cities repelled or oppressed him; even luminous Paris soon filled him with weariness. It was the first foreign city in which he made a long sojourn. French art, as reflecting the aesthetic thought of the most gifted of European races, surprised him much, but charmed him not at all. What surprised him especially were its studies of the nude, in which he recognized only an open confession of the one human weakness which, next to disloyalty or cowardice, his stoical training had taught him to most despise. Modern French literature gave him other reasons for astonishment. He could little comprehend the amazing art of the story-teller; the worth of the workmanship in itself was not visible to him; and if he could have been made to understand it as a European understands, he would have remained none the less convinced that such application of genius to production signified social depravity. And gradually, in the luxurious life of the capital itself, he found proof for the belief suggested to him by the art and the literature of the period. He visited the pleasure-resorts, the theatres, the opera; he saw with the eyes of an ascetic and a soldier, and wondered why the Western conception of the worth of life differed so little from the Far-Eastern conception of folly and of effeminacy. He saw fashionable balls, and exposures de rigueur intolerable to the Far-Eastern sense of modesty, —artistically calculated to suggest what would cause a Japanese woman to die of shame; and he wondered at criticisms he had heard about the natural, modest, healthy half-nudity of Japanese toiling under a summer sun. He saw cathedrals and churches in vast number, and near to them the palaces of vice, and establishments enriched by the stealthy sale of artistic obscenities. He listened to sermons by great preachers; and he heard blasphemies against all faith and love by priest—haters. He saw the circles of wealth, and the circles of poverty, and the abysses underlying both. The "restraining influence" of religion he did not see. That world had no faith. It was a world of mockery and masquerade and pleasure-seeking selfishness, ruled not by religion, but by police; a world into which it were not good that a man should be born.

England, more sombre, more imposing, more formidable furnished him with other problems to consider. He studied her wealth, forever growing, and the nightmares of squalor forever multiplying in the shadow of it. He saw the vast ports gorged with the riches of a hundred lands, mostly plunder; and knew the English still like their forefathers, a race of prey; and thought of the fate of her millions if she should find herself for even a single month unable to compel other races to feed them. He saw the harlotry and drunkenness that make night hideous in the world's greatest city; and he marveled at the conventional hypocrisy that pretends not to see, and at the religion that utters thanks for existing conditions, and at the ignorance that sends missionaries where they are not needed, and at the enormous charities that help disease and vice to propagate their kind. He saw also the declaration of a great Englishman(1) who had traveled in many countries that one tenth of the population of England were professional criminals or paupers. And this in spite of the myriads of churches, and the incomparable multiplication of laws! Certainly English civilization showed less than any other the pretended power of that religion which he had been taught to believe the inspiration of progress. English streets told him another story: there were no such sights to be seen in the streets of Buddhist cities. No: this civilization signified a perpetual wicked struggle between the simple and the cunning, the feeble and the strong; force and craft combining to thrust weakness into a yawning and visible hell. Never in Japan had there been even the sick dream of such conditions. Yet the merely material and intellectual results of those conditions he could not but confess to be astonishing; and though he saw evil beyond all he could have imagined possible, he also saw much good, among both poor and rich. The stupendous riddle of it all, the countless contradictions, were above his powers of interpretation.

He liked the English people better than the people of other countries he had visited; and the manners of the English gentry impressed him as not unlike those of the Japanese samurai. Behind their formal coldness he could discern immense capacities of friendship and enduring kindness,—kindness he experienced more than once; the depth of emotional power rarely wasted; and the high courage that had won the dominion of half a world. But ere he left England for America, to study a still vaster field of human achievement, mere differences of nationality had ceased to interest him: they were blurred out of visibility in his growing perception of Occidental civilization as one amazing whole, everywhere displaying—whether through imperial, monarchical, or democratic forms—the working of the like merciless necessities with the like astounding results, and everywhere based on ideas totally the reverse of Far-Eastern ideas. Such civilization he could estimate only as one having no single emotion in harmony with it,—as one finding nothing to love while dwelling in its midst, and nothing to regret in the hour of leaving it forever. It was as far away from his soul as the life of another planet under another sun. But he could understand its cost in terms of human pain, feel the menace of its weight, and divine the prodigious range of its intellectual power. And he hated it,—hated its tremendous and perfectly calculated mechanism; hated its utilitarian stability; hated its conventions, its greed, its blind cruelty, its huge hypocrisy, the foulness of its want and the insolence of its wealth. Morally, it was monstrous; conventionally, it was brutal. Depths of degradation unfathomable it had shown him, but no ideals equal to the ideals of his youth. It was all one great wolfish struggle;—and that so much real goodness as he had found in it could exist, seemed to him scarcely less than miraculous. The real sublimities of the Occident were intellectual only; far steep cold heights of pure knowledge, below whose perpetual snow-line emotional ideals die. Surely the old Japanese civilization of benevolence and duty was incomparably better in its comprehension of happiness, in its moral ambitions, its larger faith, its joyous courage, its simplicity and unselfishness, its sobriety and contentment. Western superiority was not ethical. It lay in forces of intellect developed through suffering incalculable, and used for the destruction of the weak by the strong.

And, nevertheless, that Western science whose logic he knew to be irrefutable assured him of the larger and larger expansion of the power of that civilization, as of an irresistible, inevitable, measureless inundation of world-pain. Japan would have to learn the new forms of action, to master the new forms of thought, or to perish utterly. There was no other alternative. And then the doubt of all doubts came to him, the question which all the sages have had to face: *Is the universe moral?* To that question Buddhism had given the deepest answer.

But whether moral or immoral the cosmic process, as measured by infinitesimal human emotion, one conviction remained with him that no logic could impair: the certainty that man should pursue the highest moral ideal with all his power to the unknown end, even though the suns in their courses should fight against him. The necessities of Japan would oblige her to master foreign science, to adopt much from the material civilization of her enemies; but the same necessities could not compel her to cast bodily away her ideas of right and wrong, of duty and of honor. Slowly a purpose shaped itself in his mind,—a purpose which was to make him in after years a leader and a teacher: to strive with all his strength for the conservation of all that was best in the ancient life, and to fearlessly oppose further introduction of anything not essential to national self-preservation, or helpful to national, self-development. Fail he well might, and without shame; but he could hope at least to save something of worth from the drift of wreckage. The wastefulness of Western life had impressed him more

It was through the transparent darkness of a cloudless April morning, a little before sunrise, that he saw again the mountains of his native land,—far lofty sharpening sierras, towering violet-black out of the circle of an inky sea. Behind the steamer which was bearing him back from exile the horizon was slowly filling with rosy flame. There were some foreigners already on deck, eager to obtain the first and fairest view of Fuji from the Pacific;—for the first sight of Fuji at dawn is not to be forgotten in this life or the next. They watched the long procession of the ranges, and looked over the jagged looming into the deep night, where stars were faintly burning still,—and they could not see Fuji. "Ah!" laughed an officer they questioned, "you are looking too low! higher up—much higher!" Then they looked up, up, up into the heart of the sky, and saw the mighty summit pinkening like a wondrous phantom lotos-bud in the flush of the coming day: a spectacle that smote them dumb. Swiftly the eternal snow yellowed into gold, then whitened as the sun reached out beams to it over the curve of the world, over the shadowy ranges, over the very stars, it seemed; for the giant base remained viewless. And the night fled utterly; and soft blue light bathed all the hollow heaven; and colors awoke from sleep; —and before the gazers there opened the luminous bay of Yokohama, with the sacred peak, its base ever invisible, hanging above all like a snowy ghost in the arch of the infinite day.

Still in the wanderer's ears the words rang, "*Ah! you are looking too low! —higher up—much higher!*"—making vague rhythm with an immense, irresistible emotion swelling at his heart. Then everything dimmed: he saw neither Fuji above, nor the nearing hills below, changing their vapory blue to green, nor the crowding of the ships in the bay; nor anything of the modern Japan; he saw the Old. The land-wind, delicately scented with odors of spring, rushed to him, touched his blood, and startled from long-closed cells of memory the shades of all that he had once abandoned and striven to forget. He saw the faces of his dead: he knew their voices over the graves of the years. Again he was a very little boy in his father's yashiki, wandering from luminous room to room, playing in sunned spaces where leaf-shadows trembled on the matting, or gazing into the soft green dreamy peace of the landscape garden. Once more he felt the light touch of his mother's hand guiding his little steps to the place of morning worship, before the household shrine, before the tablets of the ancestors; and the lips of the man murmured again, with sudden new-found meaning, the simple prayer of the child.

XI

IN THE TWILIGHT OF THE GODS

"Do you know anything about josses?"

"Josses?"

"Yes; idols, Japanese idols,—josses."

"Something," I answered, "but not very much."

"Well, come, and look at my collection, won't you? I've been collecting josses for twenty years, and I've got some worth seeing. They're not for sale, though,—except to the British Museum."

I followed the curio dealer through the bric-a-brac of his shop, and across a paved yard into an unusually large go-down(1). Like all go-downs it was dark: I could barely discern a stairway sloping up through gloom. He paused at the foot.

"You'll be able to see better in a moment," he said. "I had this place built expressly for them; but now it is scarcely big enough. They're all in the second story. Go right up; only be careful,—the steps are bad."

I climbed, and reached a sort of gloaming, under a very high roof, and found myself face to face with the gods.

In the dusk of the great go-down the spectacle was more than weird: it was apparitional. Arhats and Buddhas and Bodhisattvas, and the shapes of a mythology older than they, filled all the shadowy space; not ranked by hierarchies, as in a temple, but mingled without order, as in a silent panic. Out of the wilderness of multiple heads and broken aureoles and hands uplifted in menace or in prayer,—a shimmering confusion of dusty gold half lighted by cobwebbed air-holes in the heavy walls,—I could at first discern little; then, as the dimness cleared, I began to distinguish personalities. I saw Kwannon, of many forms; Jizo, of many names; Shaka, Yakushi, Amida, the Buddhas and their disciples. They were very old; and their art was not all of Japan, nor of any one place or time: there were shapes from Korea, China, India,—treasures brought over sea in the rich days of the early Buddhist missions. Some were seated upon lotos-flowers, the lotos-flowers of the Apparitional Birth. Some rode leopards, tigers, lions, or monsters mystical,—typifying lightning, typifying death. One, triple-headed and many-handed, sinister and splendid, seemed moving through the gloom on a throne of gold, uplifted by a phalanx of elephants. Fudo I saw, shrouded and shrined in fire, and Maya-Fujin, riding her celestial peacock; and strangely mingling with these Buddhist visions, as in the anachronism of a Limbo, armored effigies of Daimyo and images of the Chinese sages. There were huge forms of wrath, grasping thunderbolts, and rising to the roof: the Deva-kings, like impersonations of hurricane power; the Ni-O, guardians of long-vanished temple gates. Also there were forms voluptuously feminine: the light grace of the limbs folded within their lotos-cups, the suppleness of the fingers numbering the numbers of the Good Law, were ideals possibly inspired in some forgotten tune by the charm of an Indian dancing-girl. Shelved against the naked brickwork above, I could perceive multitudes of lesser shapes: demon figures with eyes that burned through the dark like the eyes of a black cat, and figures half man, half bird, winged and beaked like eagles,—the *Tengu* of Japanese fancy.

"Well?" queried the curio dealer, with a chuckle of satisfaction at my evident surprise.

"It is a very great collection," I responded.

He clapped his hand on my shoulder, and exclaimed triumphantly in my ear, "Cost me fifty thousand dollars."

But the images themselves told me how much more was their cost to forgotten piety, notwithstanding the cheapness of artistic labor in the East. Also they told me of the dead millions whose pilgrim feet had worn hollow the steps leading to their shrines, of the buried mothers who used to suspend little baby-dresses before their altars, of the generations of children taught to murmur prayers to them, of the countless sorrows and hopes confided to them. Ghosts of the worship of centuries had followed them into exile; a thin, sweet odor of incense haunted the dusty place.

"What would you call that?" asked the voice of the curio dealer. "I've been told it's the best of the lot."

He pointed to a figure resting upon a triple golden lotos,—Avalokitesvara: she *"who looketh down above the sound of prayer."… Storms and hate give way to her name. Fire is quenched by her name. Demons vanish at the sound of her name. By her name one may stand firm in the sky, like a sun....* The delicacy of the limbs, the tenderness of the smile, were dreams of the Indian paradise.

"It is a Kwannon," I made reply, "and very beautiful."

"Somebody will have to pay me a very beautiful price for it," he said, with a shrewd wink. "It cost me enough! As a rule, though, I get these things pretty cheap. There are few people who care to buy them, and they have to be sold privately, you know: that gives me an advantage. See that Jizo in the corner,—the big black fellow? What is it?"

"Emmei-Jizo," I answered,—"Jizo, the giver of long life. It must be very old."

"Well," he said, again taking me by the shoulder, "the man from whom I got that piece was put in prison for selling it to me."

Then he burst into a hearty laugh,—whether at the recollection of his own cleverness in the transaction, or at the unfortunate simplicity of the person who had sold the statue contrary to law, I could not decide.

"Afterwards," he resumed, "they wanted to get it back again, and offered me more, than I had given for it. But I held on. I don't know everything about josses, but I do know what they are worth. There isn't another idol like that in the whole country. The British Museum will be glad to get it."

"When do you intend to offer the collection to the British Museum?" I presumed to ask.

"Well, I first want to get up a show," he replied. "There's money to be made by a show of josses in London. London people never saw anything like this in their lives. Then the church folks help that sort of a show, if you manage them properly: it advertises the missions. 'Heathen idols from Japan!'... How do you like the baby?"

I was looking at a small gold-colored image of a naked child, standing, one tiny hand pointing upward, and the other downward, —representing the Buddha newly born. *Sparkling with light he came from the womb, as when the Sun first rises in the east.... Upright he took deliberately seven steps; and the prints of his feet upon the ground remained burning as seven stars. And he spake with clearest utterance, saying, "This birth is a Buddha birth. Re-birth is not for me. Only this last time am I born for the salvation of all on earth and in heaven."*

"That is what they call a Tanjo-Shaka," I said. "It looks like bronze."

"Bronze it is," he responded, tapping it with his knuckles to make the metal ring. "The bronze alone is worth more than the price I paid."

I looked at the four Devas whose heads almost touched the roof, and thought of the story of their apparition told in the Mahavagga. *On a beautiful night the Four Great Kings entered the holy grove, filling all the place with light; and having respectfully saluted the Blessed One, they stood in the four directions, like four great firebrands.*

"How did you ever manage to get those big figures upstairs?" I asked.

"Oh, hauled them up! We've got a hatchway. The real trouble was getting them here by train. It was the first railroad trip they ever made.... But look at these here: they will make the sensation of the show!"

I looked, and saw two small wooden images, about three feet high.

"Why do you think they will make a sensation?" I inquired innocently.

"Don't you see what they are? They date from the time of the persecutions. *Japanese devils trampling on the Cross!*"

They were small temple guardians only; but their feet rested upon X-shaped supports.

"Did any person tell you these were devils trampling on the cross?" I made bold to ask.

"What else are they doing?" he answered evasively. "Look at the crosses under their feet!"

"But they are not devils," I insisted; "and those cross-pieces were put under their feet simply to give equilibrium."

He said nothing, but looked disappointed; and I felt a little sorry for him. *Devils trampling on the Cross*, as a display line in some London poster announcing the arrival of "josses from Japan," might certainly have been relied on to catch the public eye.

"This is more wonderful," I said, pointing to a beautiful group, —Maya with the infant Buddha issuing from her side, according to tradition. *Painlessly the Bodhisattva was born from her right side. It was the eighth day of the fourth moon.*

"That's bronze, too," he remarked, tapping it. "Bronze josses are getting rare. We used to buy them up and sell them for old metal. Wish I'd kept some of them! You ought to have seen the bronzes, in those days, coming in from the temples,—bells and vases and josses! That was the time we tried to buy the Daibutsu at Kamakura."

"For old bronze?" I queried.

"Yes. We calculated the weight of the metal, and formed a syndicate. Our first offer was thirty thousand. We could have made a big profit, for there's a good deal of gold and silver in that work. The priests wanted to sell, but the people wouldn't let them."

"It's one of the world's wonders," I said. "Would you really have broken it up?"

"Certainly. Why not? What else could you do with it?… That one there looks just like a Virgin Mary, doesn't it?"

He pointed to the gilded image of a female clasping a child to her breast.

"Yes," I replied; "but it is Kishibojin, the goddess who loves little children."

"People talk about idolatry," he went on musingly. "I've seen things like many of these in Roman Catholic chapels. Seems to me religion is pretty much the same the world over."

"I think you are right," I said.

"Why, the story of Buddha is like the story of Christ, isn't it?"

"To some degree," I assented.

"Only, he wasn't crucified."

I did not answer; thinking of the text, *In all the world there is not one spot even so large as a mustard-seed where he has not surrendered his body for the sake of creatures*. Then it suddenly seemed to me that this was absolutely true. For the Buddha of the deeper Buddhism is not Gautama, nor yet any one Tathagata, but simply the divine in man. Chrysalides of the infinite we all are: each contains a ghostly Buddha, and the millions are but one. All humanity is potentially the Buddha-to-come, dreaming through the ages in Illusion; and the teacher's smile will make beautiful the world again when selfishness shall die. Every noble sacrifice brings nearer the hour of his awakening; and who may justly doubt—remembering the myriads of the centuries of man—that even now there does not remain one place on earth where life has not been freely given for love or duty?

I felt the curio dealer's hand on my shoulder again.

"At all events," he cried in a cheery tone, "they'll be appreciated in the British Museum—eh?"

"I hope so. They ought to be."

Then I fancied them immured somewhere in that vast necropolis of dead gods, under the gloom of a pea-soup-fog, chambered with forgotten divinities of Egypt or Babylon, and trembling faintly at the roar of London, —all to what end? Perhaps to aid another Alma Tadema to paint the beauty of another vanished civilization; perhaps to assist the illustration of an English Dictionary of Buddhism; perhaps to inspire some future laureate with a metaphor startling as Tennyson's figure of the "oiled and curled Assyrian bull." Assuredly they would not be preserved in vain. The thinkers of a less conventional and selfish era would teach new reverence for them. Each eidolon shaped by human faith remains the shell of a truth eternally divine, and even the shell itself may hold a ghostly power. The soft serenity, the passionless tenderness, of these Buddha faces might yet give peace of soul to a West weary of creeds transformed into conventions, eager for the coming of another teacher to proclaim, "*I have the same feeling for the high as for the low, for the moral as for the immoral, for the depraved as for the virtuous, for those holding sectarian views and false opinions as for those whose beliefs are good and true."*

(1) A name given to fireproof storehouses in the open ports of the Far East. The word is derived from the Malay gadong.

XII

THE IDEA OF PRE-EXISTENCE

"If A Bikkhu should desire, O brethren, to call to mind his various temporary states in days gone by—such as one birth, two births, three, four, five, ten, twenty, thirty, fifty, one hundred, or one thousand, or one hundred thousand births,—in all their modes and all their details, let him be devoted to quietude of heart,—let him look through things, let him be much alone."
—Akankheyya Sutta.

I

Were I to ask any reflecting Occidental, who had passed some years in the real living atmosphere of Buddhism, what fundamental idea especially differentiates Oriental modes of thinking from our own, I am sure he would answer: "The Idea of Pre-existence." It is this idea, more than any other, which permeates the whole mental being of the Far East. It is universal as the wash of air: it colors every emotion; it influences, directly or indirectly, almost every act. Its symbols are perpetually visible, even in details of artistic decoration; and hourly by day or night, some echoes of its language float uninvited to the ear. The utterances of the people,—their household sayings, their proverbs, their pious or profane exclamations, their confessions of sorrow, hope, joy, or despair,—are all informed with it. It qualifies equally the expression of hate or the speech of affection; and the term *ingwa*, or *innen*,—meaning karma as inevitable retribution, —comes naturally to every lip as an interpretation, as a consolation, or as a reproach. The peasant toiling up some steep road, and feeling the weight of his handcart straining every muscle, murmurs patiently: "Since this is ingwa, it must be suffered." Servants disputing, ask each other, "By reason of what ingwa must I now dwell with such a one as you?" The incapable or vicious man is reproached with his ingwa; and the misfortunes of the wise or the virtuous are explained by the same Buddhist word. The law-breaker confesses his crime, saying: "That which I did I knew to be wicked when doing; but my ingwa was stronger than my heart." Separated lovers seek death under the belief that their union in this life is banned by the results of their sins in a former one; and, the victim of an injustice tries to allay his natural anger by the self-assurance that he is expiating some forgotten fault which had to, be expiated in the eternal order of things…. So likewise even the commonest references to a spiritual future imply the general creed of a spiritual past. The mother warns her little ones at play about the effect of wrong-doing upon their future births, as the children of other parents. The pilgrim or the street-beggar accepts your alms with the prayer that your next birth may be fortunate. The aged *inkyo*, whose sight and hearing begin to fail, talks cheerily of the impending change that is to provide him with a fresh young body. And the expressions *Yakusoku*, signifying the Buddhist idea of necessity; *mae no yo*, the last life; *akirame*, resignation, recur as frequently in Japanese common parlance as do the words "right" and "wrong" in English popular speech.

After long dwelling in this psychological medium, you find that it has penetrated your own thought, and has effected therein various changes. All concepts of life implied by the idea of preexistence,—all those beliefs which, however sympathetically studied, must at first have seemed more than strange to you,— finally lose that curious or fantastic character with which novelty once invested them, and present themselves under a perfectly normal aspect. They explain so many things so well as even to look rational; and quite rational some assuredly are when measured by the scientific thought of the nineteenth century. But to judge them fairly, it is first necessary to sweep the mind clear of all Western ideas of metempsychosis. For there is no resemblance between the old Occidental conceptions of soul—the Pythagorean or the Platonic, for example—and the Buddhist conception; and it is precisely because of this unlikeness that the Japanese beliefs prove themselves reasonable. The profound difference between old-fashioned Western thought and Eastern thought in this regard is, that for the Buddhist the conventional soul—the single, tenuous, tremulous, transparent inner man, or ghost—does not exist. The Oriental Ego is not individual. Nor is it* even a definitely numbered multiple like the Gnostic soul. It is an aggregate or composite of inconceivable complexity,—the concentrated sum of the creative thinking of previous lives beyond all reckoning.

II

The interpretative power of Buddhism, and the singular accord of its theories with the facts of modern science, appear especially in that domain of psychology whereof Herbert Spencer has been the greatest of all explorers. No small part of our psychological life is composed of feelings which Western theology never could explain. Such are those which cause the still speechless infant to cry at the sight of certain faces, or to smile at the sight of others. Such are those instantaneous likes or dislikes experienced on meeting strangers, those repulsions or attractions called "first impressions," which intelligent children are prone to announce with alarming frankness, despite all assurance that "people must not be judged by appearances": a doctrine no child in his heart believes. To call these feelings instinctive or intuitive, in the theological meaning of instinct or intuition, explains nothing at all—merely cuts off inquiry into the mystery of life, just like the special creation hypothesis. The idea that a personal impulse or emotion might be more than individual, except through demoniacal possession, still seems to old-fashioned orthodoxy a monstrous heresy. Yet it is now certain that most of our deeper feelings are superindividual,—both those which we classify as passional, and those which we call sublime. The individuality of the amatory passion is absolutely denied by science; and what is true of love at first sight is also true of hate: both are superindividual. So likewise are those vague impulses to wander which come and go with spring, and those vague depressions experienced in autumn,—survivals, perhaps, from an epoch in which human migration followed the course of the seasons, or even from an era preceding the apparition of man. Superindividual also those emotions felt by one who, after having passed the greater part of a life on plain or prairies, first looks upon a range of snow-capped peaks; or the sensations of some dweller in the interior of a continent when he first beholds the ocean, and hears its eternal thunder. The delight, always toned with awe, which the sight of a stupendous landscape evokes; Or that speechless admiration, mingled with melancholy inexpressible, which the splendor of a tropical sunset creates,—never can be interpreted by individual experience. Psychological analysis has indeed shown these emotions to be prodigiously complex, and interwoven with personal experiences of many kinds; but in either case the deeper wave of feeling is never individual: it is a surging up from that ancestral sea of life out of which we came. To the same psychological category possibly belongs likewise a peculiar feeling which troubled men's minds long before the time of Cicero, and troubles them even more betimes in our own generation,—the feeling of having already seen a place really visited for the first time. Some strange air of familiarity about the streets of a foreign town, or the forms of a foreign landscape, comes to the mind with a sort of soft weird shock, and leaves one vainly ransacking memory for interpretations. Occasionally, beyond question, similar sensations are actually produced by the revival or recombination of former relations in consciousness; but there would seem to be many which remain wholly mysterious when we attempt to explain them by individual experience.

Even in the most common of our sensations there are enigmas never to be solved by those holding the absurd doctrine that all feeling and cognition belong to individual experience, and that the mind of the child newly-born is a *tabula rasa.* The pleasure excited by the perfume of a flower, by certain shades of color, by certain tones of music; the involuntary loathing or fear aroused by the first sight of dangerous or venomous life; even the nameless terror of dreams,—are all inexplicable upon the old-fashioned soul-hypothesis. How deeply-reaching into the life of the race some of these sensations are, such as the pleasure in odors and in colors, Grant Allen has most effectively suggested in his "Physiological Aesthetics," and in his charming treatise on the Color-Sense. But long before these were written, his teacher, the greatest of all psychologists, had clearly proven that the experience-hypothesis was utterly inadequate to account for many classes of psychological phenomena. "If possible," observes Herbert Spencer, "it is even more at fault in respect to the emotions than to the cognitions. The doctrine that all the desires, all the sentiments, are generated by the experiences of the individual, is so glaringly at variance with facts that I cannot but wonder how any one should ever have ventured to entertain it." It was Mr. Spencer, also, who showed us that words like "instinct," "intuition," have no true signification in the old sense; they must hereafter be used in a very different one. Instinct, in the language of modern psychology, means "organized memory," and memory itself is "incipient instinct,"—the sum of impressions to be inherited by the next succeeding individual in the chain of life. Thus science recognizes inherited memory:

not in the ghostly signification of a remembering of the details of former lives, but as a minute addition to psychological life accompanied by minute changes in the structure of the inherited nervous system. "The human brain is an organized register of infinitely numerous experiences received during the evolution of life, or rather, during the evolution of that series of organisms through which the human organism has been reached. The effects of the most uniform and frequent of these experiences have been successively bequeathed, principal and interest; and have slowly amounted to that high intelligence which lies latent in the brain of the infant—which the infant in after-life exercises and perhaps strengthens or further complicates—and which, with minute additions, it bequeaths to future generations(1)." Thus we have solid physiological ground for the idea of pre-existence and the idea of a multiple Ego. It is incontrovertible that in every individual brain is looked up the inherited memory of the absolutely inconceivable multitude of experiences received by all the brains of which it is the descendant. But this scientific assurance of self in the past is uttered in no materialistic sense. Science is the destroyer of materialism: it has proven matter incomprehensible; and it confesses the mystery of mind insoluble, even while obliged to postulate an ultimate unit of sensation. Out of the units of simple sensation, older than we by millions of years, have undoubtedly been built up all the emotions and faculties of man. Here Science, in accord with Buddhism, avows the Ego composite, and, like Buddhism, explains the psychical riddles of the present by the psychical experiences of the past.

(1) Principles of Psychology: "The Feelings."

III

To many persons it must seem that the idea of Soul as an infinite multiple would render impossible any idea of religion in the Western sense; and those unable to rid themselves of old theological conceptions doubtless imagine that even in Buddhist countries, and despite the evidence of Buddhist texts, the faith of the common people is really based upon the idea of the soul as a single entity. But Japan furnishes remarkable proof to the contrary. The uneducated common people, the poorest country-folk who have never studied Buddhist metaphysics, believe the self composite. What is even more remarkable is that in the primitive faith, Shinto, a kindred doctrine exists; and various forms of the belief seem to characterize the thought of the Chinese and of the Koreans. All these peoples of the Far East seem to consider the soul compound; whether in the Buddhist sense, or in the primitive sense represented by Shinto (a sort of ghostly multiplying by fission), or in the fantastic sense elaborated by Chinese astrology. In Japan I have fully satisfied myself that the belief is universal. It is not necessary to quote here from the Buddhist texts, because the common or popular beliefs, and not the philosophy of a creed, can alone furnish evidence that religious fervor is compatible and consistent with the notion of a composite soul. Certainly the Japanese peasant does not think the psychical Self nearly so complex a thing as Buddhist philosophy considers it, or as Western science proves it to be. *But he thinks of himself as multiple.* The struggle within him between impulses good and evil he explains as a conflict between the various ghostly wills that make up his Ego; and his spiritual hope is to disengage his better self or selves from his worse selves,—Nirvana, or the supreme bliss, being attainable only through the survival of the best within him. Thus his religion appears to be founded upon a natural perception of psychical evolution not nearly so remote from scientific thought as are those conventional notions of soul held by our common people at home. Of course his ideas on these abstract subjects are vague and unsystematized; but their general character and tendencies are unmistakable; and there can be no question whatever as to the earnestness of his faith, or as to the influence of that faith upon his ethical life.

Wherever belief survives among the educated classes, the same ideas obtain definition and synthesis. I may cite, in example, two selections from compositions, written by students aged respectively twenty-three and twenty-six. I might as easily cite a score; but the following will sufficiently indicate what I mean:—

"Nothing is more foolish than to declare the immortality of the soul. The soul is a compound; and though its elements be eternal, we know they can never twice combine in exactly the same way. All compound things must change their character and their conditions."

"Human life is composite. A combination of energies make the soul. When a man dies his soul may either remain unchanged, or be changed according to that which it combines with. Some philosophers say the soul is immortal; some, that it is mortal. They are both right. The soul is mortal or immortal according to the change of the combinations composing it. The elementary energies from which the soul is formed are, indeed, eternal; but the nature of the soul is determined by the character of the combinations into which those energies enter."

Now the ideas expressed in these compositions will appear to the Western reader, at first view, unmistakably atheistic. Yet they are really compatible with the sincerest and deepest faith. It is the use of the English word "soul," not understood at all as we understand it, which creates the false impression. "Soul," in the sense used by the young writers, means an almost infinite combination of both good and evil tendencies,—a compound doomed to disintegration not only by the very fact of its being a compound, but also by the eternal law of spiritual progress.

IV

That the idea, which has been for thousands of years so vast a factor in Oriental thought-life, should have failed to develop itself in the West till within, our own day, is sufficiently explained by Western theology. Still, it would not be correct to say that theology succeeded in rendering the notion of pre-existence absolutely repellent to Occidental minds. Though Christian doctrine, holding each soul specially created out of nothing to fit each new body, permitted no avowed beliefs in pre-existence, popular common-sense recognized a contradiction of dogma in the phenomena of heredity. In the same way, while theology decided animals to be mere automata, moved by a sort of incomprehensible machinery called instinct, the people generally recognized that animals had reasoning powers. The theories of instinct and of intuition held even a generation ago seem utterly barbarous to-day. They were commonly felt to be useless as interpretations; but as dogmas they served to check speculation and to prevent heresy. Wordsworth's "Fidelity" and his marvelously overrated "Intimations of Immortality" bear witness to the extreme timidity and crudeness of Western notions on these subjects even at the beginning of the century. The love of the dog for his master is indeed "great beyond all human estimate," but for reasons Wordsworth never dreamed about; and although the fresh sensations of childhood are certainly intimations of something much more wonderful than Wordsworth's denominational idea of immortality, his famous stanza concerning them has been very justly condemned by Mr. John Morley as nonsense. Before the decay of theology, no rational ideas of psychological inheritance, of the true nature of instinct, or of the unity of life, could possibly have forced their way to general recognition.

But with the acceptance of the doctrine of evolution, old forms of thought crumbled; new ideas everywhere arose to take the place of worn-out dogmas; and we now have the spectacle of a general intellectual movement in directions strangely parallel with Oriental philosophy. The unprecedented rapidity and multiformity of scientific progress during the last fifty years could not have failed to provoke an equally unprecedented intellectual quickening among the non-scientific. That the highest and most complex organisms have been developed from the lowest and simplest; that a single physical basis of life is the substance of the whole living world; that no line of separation can be drawn between the animal and vegetable; that the difference between life and non-life is only a difference of degree, not of kind; that matter is not less incomprehensible than mind, while both are but varying manifestations of one and the same unknown reality,—these have already become the commonplaces of the new philosophy. After the first recognition even by theology of physical evolution, it was easy to predict that the recognition of psychical evolution could not be indefinitely delayed; for the barrier erected by old dogma to keep men from looking backward had been broken down. And to-day for the student of scientific psychology the idea of pre-existence passes out of the realm of theory into the realm of fact, proving the Buddhist explanation of the universal mystery quite as plausible as any other. "None but very hasty thinkers," wrote the late Professor Huxley, "will reject it on the ground of inherent absurdity. Like the doctrine of evolution itself, that of transmigration has its roots in the world of reality; and it may claim such support as the great argument from analogy is capable of supplying(1)."

Now this support, as given by Professor Huxley, is singularly strong. It offers us no glimpse of a single soul flitting from darkness to light, from death to rebirth, through myriads of millions of years; but it leaves the main idea of pre-existence almost exactly in the form enunciated by the Buddha himself. In the Oriental doctrine, the psychical personality, like the individual body, is an aggregate doomed to disintegration By psychical personality I mean here that which distinguishes mind from mind,—the "me" from the "you": that which we call self. To Buddhism this is a temporary composite of illusions. What makes it is the karma. What reincarnates is the karma,—the sum-total of the acts and thoughts of countless anterior existences,—each existences,—each one of which, as an integer in some great spiritual system of addition and subtraction, may affect all the rest. Like a magnetism, the karma is transmitted from form to form, from phenomenon to phenomenon, determining conditions by combinations. The ultimate mystery of the concentrative and creative effects of karma the Buddhist acknowledges to be inscrutable; but the cohesion of effects he declares to be produced by tanha, the desire of life, corresponding to what Schopenhauer called the "will" to live. Now we find in Herbert Spencer's "Biology" a curious parallel for this idea. He explains the transmission of tendencies, and their variations, by a theory of polarities,—polarities of the physiological unit between this theory of polarities and the Buddhist theory of tanha, the difference is much less striking than the resemblance. Karma or heredity, tanha or polarity, are inexplicable as to their ultimate nature: Buddhism and Science are here at one. The fact worthy of attention is that both recognize the same phenomena under different names.

(1) Evolution and Ethics, p.61 (ed 1894).

V

The prodigious complexity of the methods by which Science has arrived at conclusions so strangely in harmony with the ancient thought of the East, may suggest the doubt whether those conclusions could ever be made clearly comprehensible to the mass of Western minds. Certainly it would seem that just as the real doctrines of Buddhism can be taught to the majority of believers through forms only, so the philosophy of science can be communicated to the masses through suggestion only,—suggestion of such facts, or arrangements of fact, as must appeal to any naturally intelligent mind. But the history of scientific progress assures the efficiency of this method; and there is no strong reason for the supposition that, because the processes of the higher science remain above the mental reach of the unscientific classes, the conclusions of that science will not be generally accepted. The dimensions and weights of planets; the distances and the composition of stars; the law of gravitation; the signification of heat, light, and color; the nature of sound, and a host of other scientific discoveries, are familiar to thousands quite ignorant of the details of the methods by which such knowledge was obtained. Again we have evidence that every great progressive movement of science during the century has been followed by considerable modifications of popular beliefs. Already the churches, though clinging still to the hypothesis of a specially-created soul, have accepted the main doctrine of physical evolution; and neither fixity of belief nor intellectual retrogression can be rationally expected in the immediate future. Further changes of religious ideas are to be looked for; and it is even likely that they will be effected rapidly rather than slowly. Their exact nature, indeed, cannot be predicted; but existing intellectual tendencies imply that the doctrine of psychological evolution must be accepted, though not at once so as to set any final limit to ontological speculation; and that the whole conception of the Ego will be eventually transformed through the consequently developed idea of pre-existence.

VI

More detailed consideration of these probabilities may be ventured. They will not, perhaps, be acknowledged as probabilities by persons who regard science as a destroyer rather than a modifier. But such thinkers forget that religious feeling is something infinitely more profound than dogma; that it survives all gods and all forms of creed; and that it only widens and deepens and gathers power with intellectual expansion. That as mere doctrine religion will ultimately pass away is a conclusion to which the study of evolution leads; but that religion as feeling, or even as faith in the unknown power shaping equally a brain or a constellation, can ever utterly die, is not at present conceivable. Science wars only upon erroneous interpretations of phenomena; it only magnifies the cosmic mystery, and proves that everything, however minute, is infinitely wonderful and incomprehensible. And it is this indubitable tendency of science to broaden beliefs and to magnify cosmic emotion which justifies the supposition that future modifications of Western religious ideas will be totally unlike any modifications effected in the past; that the Occidental conception of Self will orb into something akin to the Oriental conception of Self; and that all present petty metaphysical notions of personality and individuality as realities per se will be annihilated. Already the growing popular comprehension of the facts of heredity, as science teaches them, indicates the path by which some, at least, of these modifications will be reached. In the coming contest over the great question of psychological evolution, common intelligence will follow Science along the line of least resistance; and that line will doubtless be the study of heredity, since the phenomena to be considered, however in themselves uninterpretable, are familiar to general experience, and afford partial answers to countless old enigmas. It is thus quite possible to imagine a coming form of Western religion supported by the whole power of synthetic philosophy, differing from Buddhism mainly in the greater exactness of its conceptions, holding the soul as a composite, and teaching a new spiritual law resembling the doctrine of karma.

An objection to this idea will, however, immediately present itself to many minds. Such a modification of belief, it will be averred, would signify the sudden conquest and transformation of feelings by ideas. "The world," says Herbert Spencer, "is not governed by ideas, but by feelings, to which ideas serve only as guides." How are the notions of a change, such as that supposed, to be reconciled with common knowledge of existing religious sentiment in the West, and the force of religious emotionalism?

Were the ideas of pre-existence and of the soul as multiple really antagonistic to Western religious sentiment, no satisfactory answer could be made. But are they so antagonistic? The idea of pre-existence certainly is not; the Occidental mind is already prepared for it. It is true that the notion of Self as a composite, destined to dissolution, may seem little better than the materialistic idea of annihilation,—at least to those still unable to divest themselves of the old habits of thought. Nevertheless, impartial reflection will show that there is no emotional reason for dreading the disintegration of the Ego. Actually, though unwittingly, it is for this very disintegration that Christians and Buddhists alike perpetually pray. Who has not often wished to rid himself of the worse parts of his nature, of tendencies to folly or to wrong, of impulses to say or do unkind things,—of all that lower inheritance which still clings about the higher man, and weighs down his finest aspirations? Yet that of which we so earnestly desire the separation, the elimination, the death, is not less surely a part of psychological inheritance, of veritable Self, than are those younger and larger faculties which help to the realization of noble ideals. Rather than an end to be feared, the dissolution of Self is the one object of all objects to which our efforts should be turned. What no new philosophy can forbid us to hope is that the best elements of Self will thrill on to seek loftier affinities, to enter into grander and yet grander combinations, till the supreme revelation comes, and we discern, through infinite vision,—through the vanishing of all Self,—the Absolute Reality.

For while we know that even the so-called elements themselves are evolving, we have no proof that anything utterly dies. That we are is the certainty that, we have been and will be. We have survived countless evolutions, countless universes. We know that through the Cosmos all is law. No chance decides what units shall form the planetary core, or what shall feel the sun; what shall be locked in granite and basalt, or shall multiply in plant and in animal. So far as reason can venture to infer from analogy, the cosmical history of every ultimate unit, psychological or physical, is determined just as surely and as exactly as in the Buddhist doctrine of karma.

VII

The influence of Science will not be the only factor in the modification of Western religious beliefs: Oriental philosophy will certainly furnish another. Sanscrit, Chinese, and Pali scholarship, and the tireless labor of philologists in all parts of the East, are rapidly familiarizing Europe and America with all the great forms of Oriental thought; Buddhism is being studied with interest throughout the Occident; and the results of these studies are yearly showing themselves more and more definitely in the mental products of the highest culture. The schools of philosophy are not more visibly affected than the literature of the period. Proof that a reconsideration of the problem of the Ego is everywhere forcing itself upon Occidental minds, may be found not only in the thoughtful prose of the time, but even in its poetry and its romance. Ideas impossible a generation ago are changing current thought, destroying old tastes, and developing higher feelings. Creative art, working under larger inspiration, is telling what absolutely novel and exquisite sensations, what hitherto unimaginable pathos, what marvelous deepening of emotional power, may be gained in literature with the recognition of the idea of pre-existence. Even in fiction we learn that we have been living in a hemisphere only; that we have been thinking but half-thoughts; that we need a new faith to join past with future over the great parallel of the present, and so to round out our emotional world into a perfect sphere. The clear conviction that the self is multiple, however paradoxical the statement seem, is the absolutely necessary step to the vaster conviction that the many are One, that life is unity, that there is no finite, but only infinite. Until that blind pride which imagines Self unique shall have been broken down, and the feeling of self and of selfishness shall have been utterly decomposed, the knowledge of the Ego as infinite,—as the very Cosmos,—never can be reached.

Doubtless the simple emotional conviction that we have been in the past will be developed long before the intellectual conviction that the Ego as one is a fiction of selfishness. But the composite nature of Self must at last be acknowledged, though its mystery remain. Science postulates a hypothetical psychological unit as well as a hypothetical physiological unit; but either postulated entity defies the uttermost power of mathematical estimate,—seems to resolve itself into pure ghostliness. The chemist, for working purposes, must imagine an ultimate atom; but the fact of which the imagined atom is the symbol may be a force centre only,—nay, a void, a vortex, an emptiness, as in Buddhist concept. "*Form is emptiness, and emptiness is form. What is form, that is emptiness; what is emptiness, that is form. Perception and conception, name and knowledge,—all these are emptiness.*" For science and for Buddhism alike the cosmos resolves itself into a vast phantasmagoria,—a mere play of unknown and immeasurable forces. Buddhist faith, however, answers the questions "Whence?" and "Whither?" in its own fashion, and predicts in every great cycle of evolution a period of spiritual expansion in which the memory of former births returns, and all the future simultaneously opens before the vision unveiled, even to the heaven of heavens. Science here remains dumb. But her silence is the Silence of the Gnostics,—Sige, the Daughter of Depth and the Mother of Spirit.

What we may allow ourselves to believe, with the full consent of Science, is that marvelous revelations await us. Within recent time new senses and powers have been developed,—the sense of music, the ever-growing faculties of the mathematician. Reasonably it may be expected that still higher unimaginable faculties will be evolved in our descendants. Again it is known that certain mental capacities, undoubtedly inherited, develop in old age only; and the average life of the human race is steadily lengthening. With increased longevity there surely may come into sudden being, through the unfolding of the larger future brain, powers not less wonderful than the ability to remember former births. The dreams of Buddhism can scarcely be surpassed, because they touch the infinite; but who can presume to say they never will be realized?

NOTE.

It may be necessary to remind some of those kind enough to read the foregoing that the words "soul," "self," "ego," "transmigration," "heredity," although freely used by me, convey meanings entirely foreign to Buddhist philosophy, "Soul," in the English sense of the word, does not exist for the Buddhist. "Self" is an illusion, or rather a plexus of illusions. "Transmigration," as the passing of soul from one body to another, is expressly denied in Buddhist texts of unquestionable authority. It will therefore be evident that the real analogy which does exist between the doctrine of karma and the scientific facts of heredity is far from complete. Karma signifies the survival, not of the same composite individuality, but of its tendencies, which recombine to form a new composite individuality. The new being does not necessarily take even a human form: the karma does not descend from parent to child; it is independent of the line of heredity, although physical conditions of life seem to depend upon karma. The karma-being of a beggar may have rebirth in the body of a king; that of a king in the body of a beggar; yet the conditions of either reincarnation have been predetermined by the influence of karma.

It will be asked, What then is the spiritual element in each being that continues unchanged,—the spiritual kernel, so to speak, within the shell of karma,—the power that makes for righteousness? If soul and body alike are temporary composites, and the karma (itself temporary) the only source of personality, what is the worth or meaning of Buddhist doctrine? What is it that suffers by karma; what is it that lies within the illusion, —that makes progress,—that attains Nirvana? Is it not a self? Not in our sense of the word. The reality of what we call self is denied by Buddhism. That which forms and dissolves the karma; that which makes for righteousness; that which reaches Nirvana, is not our Ego in our Western sense of the word. Then what is it? It is the divine in each being. It is called in Japanese Muga-no-taiga,—the Great Self-without-selfishness. There Is no other true self. The self wrapped in illusion is called Nyorai-zo,—(Tathagata-gharba),—the Buddha yet unborn, as one in a womb. The Infinite exists potentially in every being. That is the Reality. The other self is a falsity,—-a lie,—a mirage. The doctrine of extinction refers only to the extinction of Illusions; and those sensations and feelings and thoughts, which belong to this life of the flesh alone, are the illusions which make the complex illusive self. By the total decomposition of this false self,—as by a tearing away of veils, the Infinite Vision comes. There is no "soul": the Infinite All-Soul is the only eternal principle in any being;—all the rest is dream.

What remains in Nirvana? According to one school of Buddhism potential identity in the infinite,—so that a Buddha, after having reached Nirvana, can return to earth. According to another, identity more than potential, yet not in our sense "personal." A Japanese friend says:—"I take a piece of gold, and say it is one. But this means that it produces on my visual organs a single impression. Really in the multitude of atoms composing it each atom is nevertheless distinct and separate, and independent of every other atom. In Buddhahood even so are united psychical atoms innumerable. They are one as to condition;—yet each has its own independent existence."

But in Japan the primitive religion has so affected the common class of Buddhist beliefs that it is not incorrect to speak of the Japanese "idea of self." It is only necessary that the popular Shinto idea be simultaneously considered. In Shinto we have the plainest possible evidence of the conception of soul. But this soul is a composite,—not a mere "bundle of sensations, perceptions, and volitions," like the karma-being, but a number of souls united to form one ghostly personality. A dead man's ghost may appear as one or as many. It can separate its units, each of which remains capable of a special independent action. Such separation, however, appears to be temporary, the various souls of the composite naturally cohering even after death, and reuniting after any voluntary separation. The vast mass of the Japanese people are both Buddhists and Shintoists; but the primitive beliefs concerning the self are certainly the most powerful, and in the blending of the two faiths remain distinctly recognizable. They have probably supplied to common imagination a natural and easy explanation of the difficulties of the karma-doctrine, though to what extent I am not prepared to say. Be it also observed that in the primitive as well as in the Buddhist form of belief the self is not a principle transmitted from parent to offspring,—not an inheritance always dependent upon physiological descent.

These facts will indicate how wide is the difference between Eastern ideas and our own upon the subject of the preceding essay. They will also show that any general consideration of the real analogies existing between this strange combination of Far-Eastern beliefs and the scientific thought of the nineteenth century could scarcely be made intelligible by strict philosophical accuracy in the use of terms relating to the idea of self. Indeed, there are no European words capable of rendering the exact meaning of the Buddhist terms belonging to Buddhist Idealism.

Perhaps it may be regarded as illegitimate to wander from that position so tersely enunciated by Professor Huxley in his essay on "Sensation and the Sensiferous Organs:" "In ultimate analysis it appears that a sensation is the equivalent in terms of consciousness for a mode of motion of the matter of the sensorium. But if inquiry is pushed a stage further, and the question is asked, What, then, do we know about matter and motion? there is but one reply possible. All we know about motion is that it is a name for certain changes in the relations of our visual, tactile, and muscular sensations; and all we know about matter is that it is the hypothetical substance of physical phenomena, *the assumption of which is as pure a piece of metaphysical speculation as is that of a substance of mind*." But metaphysical speculation certainly will not cease because of scientific recognition that ultimate truth is beyond the utmost possible range of human knowledge. Rather, for that very reason, it will continue. Perhaps it will never wholly cease. Without it there can be no further modification of religious beliefs, and without modifications there can be no religious progress in harmony with scientific thought. Therefore, metaphysical speculation seems to me not only justifiable, but necessary.

Whether we accept or deny a *substance* of mind; whether we imagine thought produced by the play of some unknown element through the cells of the brain, as music is made by the play of wind through the strings of a harp; whether we regard the motion itself as a special mode of vibration inherent in and peculiar to the units of the cerebral structure,—still the mystery is infinite, and still Buddhism remains a noble moral working-hypothesis, in deep accord with the aspirations of mankind and with the laws of ethical progression. Whether we believe or disbelieve in the reality of that which is called the material universe, still the ethical significance of the inexplicable laws of heredity—of the transmission of both racial and personal tendencies in the unspecialized reproductive cell—remains to justify the doctrine of karma. Whatever be that which makes consciousness, its relation to all the past and to all the future is unquestionable. Nor can the doctrine of Nirvana ever cease to command the profound respect of the impartial thinker. Science has found evidence that known substance is not less a product of evolution than mind,—that all our so-called "elements" have been evolved out of "one primary undifferentiated form of matter." And this evidence is startlingly suggestive of some underlying truth in the Buddhist doctrine of emanation and illusion,—the evolution of all forms from the Formless, of all material phenomena from immaterial Unity,—and the ultimate return of all into "that state which is empty of lusts, of malice, of dullness,—that state in which the excitements of individuality are known no more, and which is therefore designated THE VOID SUPREME."

XIII

IN CHOLERA-TIME

I

China's chief ally in the late war, being deaf and blind, knew nothing, and still knows nothing, of treaties or of peace. It followed the returning armies of Japan, invaded the victorious empire, and killed about thirty thousand people during the hot season. It is still slaying; and the funeral pyres burn continually. Sometimes the smoke and the odor come wind-blown into my garden down from the hills behind the town, just to remind me that the cost of burning an adult of my own size is eighty sen,—about half a dollar in American money at the present rate of exchange.

From the upper balcony of my house, the whole length of a Japanese street, with its rows of little shops, is visible down to the bay. Out of various houses in that street I have seen cholera-patients conveyed to the hospital,—the last one (only this morning) my neighbor across the way, who kept a porcelain shop. He was removed by force, in spite of the tears and cries of his family. The sanitary law forbids the treatment of cholera in private houses; yet people try to hide their sick, in spite of fines and other penalties, because the public cholera-hospitals are overcrowded and roughly managed, and the patients are entirely separated from all who love them. But the police are not often deceived: they soon discover unreported cases, and come with litters and coolies. It seems cruel; but sanitary law must be cruel. My neighbor's wife followed the litter, crying, until the police obliged her to return to her desolate little shop. It is now closed up, and will probably never be opened again by the owners.

Such tragedies end as quickly as they begin. The bereaved, so soon as the law allows, remove their pathetic belongings, and disappear; and the ordinary life of the street goes on, by day and by night, exactly as if nothing particular had happened. Itinerant venders, with their bamboo poles and baskets or buckets or boxes, pass the empty houses, and utter their accustomed cries; religious processions go by, chanting fragments of sutras; the blind shampooer blows his melancholy whistle; the private watchman makes his heavy staff boom upon the gutter-flags; the boy who sells confectionery still taps his drum, and sings a love-song with a plaintive sweet voice, like a girl's:—

"*You and I together*.... I remained long; yet in the moment of going I thought I had only just come.

"You and I together.... Still I think of the tea. Old or new tea of Uji it might have seemed to others; but to me it was Gyokoro tea, of the beautiful yellow of the yamabuki flower.

"You and I together.... I am the telegraph-operator; you are the one who waits the message. I send my heart, and you receive it. What care we now if the posts should fall, if the wires be broken?"

And the children sport as usual. They chase one another with screams and laughter; they dance in chorus; they catch dragon-flies and tie them to long strings; they sing burdens of the war, about cutting off Chinese heads:—

"Chan-chan bozu no Kubi wo hane!"

Sometimes a child vanishes; but the survivers continue their play. And this is wisdom.

It costs only forty-four sen to burn a child. The son of one of my neighbors was burned a few days ago. The little stones with which he used to play lie there in the sun just as he left them.... Curious, this child-love of stones! Stones are the toys not only of the children of the poor, but of all children at one period of existence: no matter how well supplied with other playthings, every Japanese child wants sometimes to play with stones. To the child-mind a stone is a marvelous thing, and ought so to be, since even to the understanding of the mathematician there can be nothing more wonderful than a common stone. The tiny urchin suspects the stone to be much more than it seems, which is an excellent suspicion; and if stupid grown-up folk did not untruthfully tell him that his plaything is not worth thinking about, he would never tire of it, and would always be finding something new and extraordinary in it. Only a very great mind could answer all a child's questions about stones.

According to popular faith, my neighbor's darling is now playing with small ghostly stones in the Dry Bed of the River of Souls, —wondering, perhaps, why they cast no shadows. The true poetry in the legend of the Sai-no-Kawara is the absolute naturalness of its principal idea,—the phantom-continuation of that play which all little Japanese children play with stones.

II

The pipe-stem seller used to make his round with two large boxes suspended from a bamboo pole balanced upon his shoulder: one box containing stems of various diameters, lengths, and colors, together with tools for fitting them into metal pipes; and the other box containing a baby, —his own baby. Sometimes I saw it peeping over the edge of the box, and smiling at the passers-by; sometimes I saw it lying, well wrapped up and fast asleep, in the bottom of the box; sometimes I saw it playing with toys. Many people, I was told, used to give it toys. One of the toys bore a curious resemblance to a mortuary tablet (ihai); and this I always observed in the box, whether the child were asleep or awake.

The other day I discovered that the pipe-stem seller had abandoned his bamboo pole and suspended boxes. He was coming up the street with a little hand-cart just big enough to hold his wares and his baby, and evidently built for that purpose in two compartments. Perhaps the baby had become too heavy for the more primitive method of conveyance. Above the cart fluttered a small white flag, bearing in cursive characters the legend *Ki-seru-rao kae* (pipe-stems exchanged), and a brief petition for "honorable help," *O-tasuke wo negaimasu.* The child seemed well and happy; and I again saw the tablet-shaped object which had so often attracted my notice before. It was now fastened upright to a high box in the cart facing the infant's bed. As I watched the cart approaching, I suddenly felt convinced that the tablet was really an ihai: the sun shone full upon it, and there was no mistaking the conventional Buddhist text. This aroused my curiosity; and I asked Manyemon to tell the pipe-stem seller that we had a number of pipes needing fresh stems,—which was true. Presently the cartlet drew up at our gate, and I went to look at it.

The child was not afraid, even of a foreign face,—a pretty boy. He lisped and laughed and held out his arms, being evidently used to petting; and while playing with him I looked closely at the tablet. It was a Shinshu ihai, bearing a woman's kaimyo, or posthumous name; and Manyemon translated the Chinese characters for me: *Revered and of good rank in the Mansion of Excellence, the thirty-first day of the third month of the twenty-eighth year of Meiji.* Meantime a servant had fetched the pipes which needed new stems; and I glanced at the face of the artisan as he worked. It was the face of a man past middle age, with those worn, sympathetic lines about the mouth, dry beds of old smiles, which give to so many Japanese faces an indescribable expression of resigned gentleness. Presently Manyemon began to ask questions; and when Manyemon asks questions, not to reply is possible for the wicked only. Sometimes behind that dear innocent old head I think I see the dawning of an aureole,—the aureole of the Bosatsu.

The pipe-stem seller answered by telling his story. Two months after the birth of their little boy, his wife had died. In the last hour of her illness she had said: "From what time I die till three full years be past I pray you to leave the child always united with the Shadow of me: never let him be separated from my ihai, so that I may continue to care for him and to nurse him— since thou knowest that he should have the breast for three years. This, my last asking, I entreat thee, do not forget." But the mother being dead, the father could not labor as he had been wont to do, and also take care of so young a child, requiring continual attention both night and day; and he was too poor to hire a nurse. So he took to selling pipe-stems, as he could thus make a little money without leaving the child even for a minute alone. He could not afford to buy milk; but he had fed the boy for more than a year with rice gruel and cane syrup.

I said that the child looked very strong, and none the worse for lack of milk.

"That," declared Manyemon, in a tone of conviction bordering on reproof, "is because the dead mother nurses him. How should he want for milk?"

And the boy laughed softly, as if conscious of a ghostly caress.

XIV

SOME THOUGHTS ABOUT ANCESTOR-WORSHIP

"For twelve leagues, Ananda, around the Sala-Grove, there is no spot in size even as the pricking of the point of the tip of a hair, which is not pervaded by powerful spirits." —The Book Of the Great Decease.

I

The truth that ancestor-worship, in various unobtrusive forms, still survives in some of the most highly civilized countries of Europe, is not so widely known as to preclude the idea that any non-Aryan race actually practicing so primitive a cult must necessarily remain in the primitive stage of religious thought. Critics of Japan have pronounced this hasty judgment;

and have professed themselves unable to reconcile the facts of her scientific progress, and the success of her advanced educational system, with the continuance of her ancestor-worship. How can the beliefs of Shinto coexist with the knowledge of modern science? How can the men who win distinction as scientific specialists still respect the household shrine or do reverence before the Shinto parish-temple? Can all this mean more than the ordered conservation of forms after the departure of faith? Is it not certain that with the further progress of education, Shinto, even as ceremonialism, must cease to exist?

Those who put such questions appear to forget that similar questions might be asked about the continuance of any Western faith, and similar doubts expressed as to the possibility of its survival for another century. Really the doctrines of Shinto are not in the least degree more irreconcilable with modern science than are the doctrines of Orthodox Christianity. Examined with perfect impartiality, I would even venture to say that they are less irreconcilable in more respects than one. They conflict less with our human ideas of justice; and, like the Buddhist doctrine of karma, they offer some very striking analogies with the scientific facts of heredity,— analogies which prove Shinto to contain an element of truth as profound as any single element of truth in any of the world's great religions. Stated in the simplest possible form, the peculiar element of truth in Shinto is the belief that the world of the living is directly governed by the world of the dead.

That every impulse or act of man is the work of a god, and that all the dead become gods, are the basic ideas of the cult. It must be remembered, however, that the term Kami, although translated by the term deity, divinity, or god, has really no such meaning as that which belongs to the English words: it has not even the meaning of those words as referring to the antique beliefs of Greece and Rome. It signifies that which is "above," "superior," "upper," "eminent," in the non-religious sense; in the religious sense it signifies a human spirit having obtained supernatural power after death. The dead are the "powers above," the "upper ones,"—the Kami. We have here a conception resembling very strongly the modern Spiritualistic notion of ghosts, only that the Shinto idea is in no true sense democratic. The Kami are ghosts of greatly varying dignity and power,—belonging to spiritual hierarchies like the hierarchies of ancient Japanese society. Although essentially superior to the living in certain respects, the living are, nevertheless, able to give them pleasure or displeasure, to gratify or to offend them,—even sometimes to ameliorate their spiritual condition. Wherefore posthumous honors are never mockeries, but realities, to the Japanese mind. During the present year(1), for example, several distinguished statesmen and soldiers were raised to higher rank immediately after their death; and I read only the other day, in the official gazette, that "His Majesty has been pleased to posthumously confer the Second Class of the Order of the Rising Sun upon Major-General Baron Yamane, who lately died in Formosa." Such imperial acts must not be regarded only as formalities intended to honor the memory of brave and patriotic men; neither should they be thought of as intended merely to confer distinction upon the family of the dead. They are essentially of Shinto, and exemplify that intimate sense of relation between the visible and invisible worlds which is the special religious characteristic of Japan among all civilized countries. To Japanese thought the dead are not less real than the living. They take part in the daily life of the people,—sharing the humblest sorrows and the humblest joys. They attend the family repasts, watch over the well-being of the household, assist and rejoice in the prosperity of their descendants. They are present at the public pageants, at all the sacred festivals of Shinto, at the military games, and at all the entertainments especially provided for them. And they are universally thought of as finding pleasure in the offerings made to them or the honors conferred upon them.

For the purpose of this little essay, it will be sufficient to consider the Kami as the spirits of the dead,—without making any attempt to distinguish such Kami from those primal deities believed to have created the land. With this general interpretation of the term Kami, we return, then, to the great Shinto idea that all the dead still dwell in the world and rule it; influencing not only the thoughts and the acts of men, but the conditions of nature. "They direct," wrote Motowori, "the changes of the seasons, the wind and the rain, the good and the bad fortunes of states and of individual men." They are, in short, the viewless forces behind all phenomena.

(1) Written in September, 1896.

II

The most interesting sub-theory of this ancient spiritualism is that which explains the impulses and acts of men as due to the influence of the dead. This hypothesis no modern thinker can declare irrational, since it can claim justification from the scientific doctrine of psychological evolution, according to which each living brain represents the structural work of innumerable dead lives,—each character a more or less imperfectly balanced sum of countless dead experiences with good and evil. Unless we deny psychological heredity, we cannot honestly deny that our impulses and feelings, and the higher capacities evolved through the feelings, have literally been shaped by the dead, and bequeathed to us by the dead; and even that the general direction of our mental activities has been determined by the power of the special tendencies bequeathed to us. In such a sense the dead are indeed our Kami and all our actions are truly influenced by them. Figuratively we may say that every mind is a world of ghosts,—ghosts incomparably more numerous than the acknowledged millions of the higher Shinto Kami and that the spectral population of one grain of brain-matter more than realizes the wildest fancies of the medieval schoolmen about the number of angels able to stand on the point of a needle. Scientifically we know that within one tiny living cell may be stored up the whole life of a race,—the sum of all the past sensation of millions of years; perhaps even (who knows?) of millions of dead planets.

But devils would not be inferior to angels in the mere power of congregating upon the point of a needle. What, of bad men and of bad acts in this theory of Shinto? Motowori made answer; "Whenever anything goes wrong in the world, it is to be attributed to the action of the evil gods called the Gods of Crookedness, whose power is so great that the Sun-Goddess and the Creator-God are sometimes powerless to restrain them; much less are human beings always able to resist their influence. The prosperity of the wicked, and the misfortunes of the good, which seem opposed to ordinary justice, are thus explained." All bad acts are due to the influence of evil deities; and evil men may become evil Kami. There are no self-contradictions in this simplest of cults(1),—nothing complicated or hard to be understood. It is not certain that all men guilty of bad actions necessarily become "gods of crookedness," for reasons hereafter to be seen; but all men, good or bad, become Kami, or influences. And all evil acts are the results of evil influences.

Now this teaching is in accord with certain facts of heredity. Our best faculties are certainly bequests from the best of our ancestors; our evil qualities are inherited from natures in which evil, or that which we now call evil, once predominated. The ethical knowledge evolved within us by civilization demands that we strengthen the high powers bequeathed us by the best experience of our dead, and diminish the force of the baser tendencies we inherit. We are under obligation to reverence and to obey our good Kami, and to strive against our gods of crookedness. The knowledge of the existence of both is old as human reason. In some form or other, the doctrine of evil and of good spirits in personal attendance upon every soul is common to most of the great religions. Our own mediaeval faith developed the idea to a degree which must leave an impress on our language for all time; yet the faith in guardian angels and tempting demons evolutionarily represents only the development of a cult once simple as the religion of the Kami. And this theory of mediaeval faith is likewise pregnant with truth. The white-winged form that whispered good into the right ear, the black shape that murmured evil into the left, do not indeed walk beside the man of the nineteenth century, but they dwell within his brain; and he knows their voices and feels their urging as well and as often as did his ancestors of the Middle Ages.

The modern ethical objection to Shinto is that both good and evil Kami are to be respected. "Just as the Mikado worshiped the gods of heaven and of earth, so his people prayed to the good gods in order to obtain blessings, and performed rites in honor of the bad gods to avert their displeasure.... As there are bad as well as good gods, it is necessary to propitiate them with offerings of agreeable food, with the playing of harps and the blowing of flutes, with singing and dancing, and with whatever else is likely to put them in good-humor(2)." As a matter of fact, in modern Japan, the evil Kami appear to receive few offerings or honors, notwithstanding this express declaration that they are to be propitiated. But it will now be obvious why the early missionaries characterized such a cult as devil-worship, —although, to Shinto imagination, the idea of a devil, in the Western meaning of the word, never took shape. The seeming weakness of the doctrine is in the teaching that evil spirits are not to be warred upon,—a teaching essentially repellent to Roman Catholic feeling. But between the evil spirits of Christian and of Shinto belief there is a vast difference. The evil Kami is only the ghost of a dead man, and is not believed to be altogether evil,—since propitiation is possible. The conception of absolute, unmixed evil is not of the Far East. Absolute evil is certainly foreign to human nature, and therefore impossible in human ghosts. The evil Kami are not devils. They are simply ghosts, who influence the passions of men; and only in this sense the deities of the passions. Now Shinto is of all religions the most natural, and therefore in certain respects the most rational. It does not consider the passions necessarily evil in themselves, but evil only according to cause, conditions, and degrees of their indulgence. Being ghosts, the gods are altogether human,—having the various good and bad qualities of men in varying proportions. The majority are good, and the sum of the influence of all is toward good rather than evil. To appreciate the rationality of this view requires a tolerably high opinion of mankind,—such an opinion as the conditions of the old society of Japan might have justified. No pessimist could profess pure Shintoism. The doctrine is optimistic; and whoever has a generous faith in humanity will have no fault to find with the absence of the idea of implacable evil from its teaching.

Now it is just in the recognition of the necessity for propitiating the evil ghosts that the ethically rational character of Shinto reveals itself. Ancient experience and modern knowledge unite in warning us against the deadly error of trying to extirpate or to paralyze certain tendencies in human nature,—tendencies which, if morbidly cultivated or freed from all restraint, lead to folly, to crime, and to countless social evils. The animal passions, the ape-and-tiger impulses, antedate human society, and are the accessories to nearly all crimes committed against it. But they cannot be killed; and they cannot be safely starved. Any attempt to extirpate them would signify also an effort to destroy some of the very highest emotional faculties with which they remain inseparably blended. The primitive impulses cannot even be numbed save at the cost of intellectual and emotional powers which give to human life all its beauty and all its tenderness, but which are, nevertheless, deeply rooted in the archaic soil of passion. The highest in us had its beginnings in the lowest. Asceticism, by warring against the natural feelings, has created monsters. Theological legislation, irrationally directed against human weaknesses, has only aggravated social disorders; and laws against pleasure have only provoked debaucheries. The history of morals teaches very plainly indeed that our bad Kami require some propitiation. The passions still remain more powerful than the reason in man, because they are incomparably older,—because they were once all-essential to self-preservation,—because they made that primal stratum of consciousness, out of which the nobler sentiments have slowly grown. Never can they be suffered to rule; but woe to whosoever would deny their immemorial rights!

(1) I am considering only the pure Shinto belief as expounded by Shinto scholars. But it may be necessary to remind the reader that both Buddhism and Shintoism are blended in Japan, not only with each other, but with Chinese ideas of various kinds. It is doubtful whether the pure Shinto ideas now exist in their original form in popular belief. We are not quite clear as to the doctrine of multiple souls in Shinto,—whether the psychical combination was originally thought of as dissolved by death. My own opinion, the result of investigation in different parts of Japan, is that the multiple soul was formerly believed to remain multiple after death.

(2) Motowori, translated by Satow.

III

Out of these primitive, but—as may now be perceived—not irrational beliefs about the dead, there have been evolved moral sentiments unknown to Western civilization. These are well worth considering, as they will prove in harmony with the most advanced conception of ethics,—and especially with that immense though yet indefinite expansion of the sense of duty which has followed upon the understanding of evolution. I do not know that we have any reason to congratulate ourselves upon the absence from our lives of the sentiments in question;—I am even inclined to think that we may yet find it morally necessary to cultivate sentiments of the same kind. One of the surprises of our future will certainly be a return to beliefs and ideas long ago abandoned upon the mere assumption that they contained no truth,—belief still called barbarous, pagan, mediaeval, by those who condemn them out of traditional habit. Year after year the researches of science afford us new proof that the savage, the barbarian, the idolater, the monk, each and all have arrived, by different paths, as near to some one point of eternal truth as any thinker of the nineteenth century. We are now learning, also, that the theories of the astrologers and of the alchemists were but partially, not totally, wrong. We have reason even to suppose that no dream of the invisible world has ever been dreamed,—that no hypothesis of the unseen has ever been imagined,—which future science will not prove to have contained some germ of reality.

Foremost among the moral sentiments of Shinto is that of loving gratitude to the past,—a sentiment having no real correspondence in our own emotional life. We know our past better than the Japanese know theirs; —we have myriads of books recording or considering its every incident and condition: but we cannot in any sense be said to love it or to feel grateful to it. Critical recognitions of its merits and of its defects;—some rare enthusiasms excited by its beauties; many strong denunciations of its mistakes: these represent the sum of our thoughts and feelings about it. The attitude of our scholarship in reviewing it is necessarily cold; that of our art, often more than generous; that of our religion, condemnatory for the most part. Whatever the point of view from which we study it, our attention is mainly directed to the work of the dead,—either the visible work that makes our hearts beat a little faster than usual while looking at it, or the results of their thoughts and deeds in relation to the society of their time. Of past humanity as unity,—of the millions long-buried as real kindred,—we either think not at all, or think only with the same sort of curiosity that we give to the subject of extinct races. We do indeed find interest in the record of some individual lives that have left large marks in history;—our emotions are stirred by the memories of great captains, statesmen, discoverers, reformers, —but only because the magnitude of that which they accomplished appeals to our own ambitions, desires, egotisms, and not at all to our altruistic sentiments in ninety-nine cases out of a hundred. The nameless dead to whom we owe most we do not trouble ourselves about,—we feel no gratitude, no love to them. We even find it difficult to persuade ourselves that the love of ancestors can possibly be a real, powerful, penetrating, life-moulding, religious emotion in any form of human society,—which it certainly is in Japan. The mere idea is utterly foreign to our ways of thinking, feeling, acting. A partial reason for this, of course, is that we have no common faith in the existence of an active spiritual relation between our ancestors and ourselves. If we happen to be irreligious, we do not believe in ghosts. If we are profoundly religious, we think of the dead as removed from us by judgment,—as absolutely separated from us during the period of our lives. It is true that among the peasantry of Roman Catholic countries there still exists a belief that the dead are permitted to return to earth once a year,—on the night of All Souls. But even according to this belief they are not considered as related to the living by any stronger bond than memory; and they are thought of,—as our collections of folk-lore bear witness,—rather with fear than love.

In Japan the feeling toward the dead is utterly different. It is a feeling of grateful and reverential love. It is probably the most profound and powerful of the emotions of the race,—that which especially directs national life and shapes national character. Patriotism belongs to it. Filial piety depends upon it. Family love is rooted in it. Loyalty is based upon it. The soldier who, to make a path for his comrades through the battle, deliberately flings away his life with a shout of "*Teikoku manzai!*"—the son or daughter who unmurmuring sacrifices all the happiness of existence for the sake, perhaps, of an undeserving or even cruel, parent; the partisan who gives up friends, family, and fortune, rather than break the verbal promise made in other years to a now poverty-stricken master; the wife who ceremoniously robes herself in white, utters a prayer, and thrusts a sword into her throat to atone for a wrong done to strangers by her husband,—all these obey the will and hear the approval of invisible witnesses. Even among the skeptical students of the new generation, this feeling survives many wrecks of faith, and the old sentiments are still uttered: "Never must we cause shame to our ancestors;" "it is our duty to give honor to our ancestors." During my former engagement as a teacher of English, it happened more than once that ignorance of the real meaning behind such phrases prompted me to change them in written composition. I would suggest, for example, that the expression, "to do honor to the memory of our ancestors," was more correct than the phrase given. I remember one day even attempting to explain why we ought not to speak of ancestors exactly as if they were living parents! Perhaps my pupils suspected me of trying to meddle with their beliefs; for the Japanese never think of an ancestor as having become "only a memory": their dead are alive.

Were there suddenly to arise within us the absolute certainty that our dead are still with us,—seeing every act, knowing our every thought, hearing each word we utter, able to feel sympathy with us or anger against us, able to help us and delighted to receive our help, able to love us and greatly needing our love,— it is quite certain that our conceptions of life and duty would be vastly changed. We should have to recognize our obligations to the past in a very solemn way. Now, with the man of the Far East, the constant presence of the dead has been a matter of conviction for thousands of years: he speaks to them daily; he tries to give them happiness; and, unless a professional criminal he never quite forgets his duty towards them. No one, says Hirata, who constantly discharges that duty, will ever be disrespectful to the gods or to his living parents. "Such a man will also be loyal to his friends, and kind and gentle with his wife and children; for the essence of this devotion is in truth filial piety." And it is in this sentiment that the secret of much strange feeling in Japanese character must be sought. Far more foreign to our world of sentiment than the splendid courage with which death is faced, or the equanimity with which the most trying sacrifices are made, is the simple deep emotion of the boy who, in the presence of a Shinto shrine never seen before, suddenly feels the tears spring to his eyes. He is conscious in that moment of what we never emotionally recognize,—the prodigious debt of the present to the past, and the duty of love to the dead.

IV

If we think a little about our position as debtors, and our way of accepting that position, one striking difference between Western and Far-Eastern moral sentiment will become manifest.

There is nothing more awful than the mere fact of life as mystery when that fact first rushes fully into consciousness. Out of unknown darkness we rise a moment into sun-light, look about us, rejoice and suffer, pass on the vibration of our being to other beings, and fall back again into darkness. So a wave rises, catches the light, transmits its motion, and sinks back into sea. So a plant ascends from clay, unfolds its leaves to light and air, flowers, seeds, and becomes clay again. Only, the wave has no knowledge; the plant has no perceptions. Each human life seems no more than a parabolic curve of motion out of earth and back to earth; but in that brief interval of change it perceives the universe. The awfulness of the phenomenon is that nobody knows anything about it. No mortal can explain this most common, yet most incomprehensible of all facts,—life in itself; yet every mortal who can think has been obliged betimes, to think about it in relation to self.

I come out of mystery;—I see the sky and the land, men and women and their works; and I know that I must return to mystery;—and merely what this means not even the greatest of philosophers—not even Mr. Herbert Spencer—can tell me. We are all of us riddles to ourselves and riddles to each other; and space and motion and time are riddles; and matter is a riddle. About the before and the after neither the newly-born nor the dead have any message for us. The child is dumb; the skull only grins. Nature has no consolation for us. Out of her formlessness issue forms which return to formlessness,—that is all. The plant becomes clay; the clay becomes a plant. When the plant turns to clay, what becomes of the vibration which was its life? Does it go on existing viewlessly, like the forces that shape spectres of frondage in the frost upon a window-pane?

Within the horizon-circle of the infinite enigma, countless lesser enigmas, old as the world, awaited the coming of man. Oedipus had to face one Sphinx; humanity, thousands of thousands,—all crouching among bones along the path of Time, and each with a deeper and a harder riddle. All the sphinxes have not been satisfied; myriads line the way of the future to devour lives yet unborn; but millions have been answered. We are now able to exist without perpetual horror because of the relative knowledge that guides us, the knowledge won out of the jaws of destruction.

All our knowledge is bequeathed knowledge. The dead have left us record of all they were able to learn about themselves and the world,—about the laws of death and life,—about things to be acquired and things to be avoided,—about ways of making existence less painful than Nature willed it,—about right and wrong and sorrow and happiness,—about the error of selfishness, the wisdom of kindness, the obligation of sacrifice. They left us information of everything they could find out concerning climates and seasons and places,—the sun and moon and stars,—the motions and the composition of the universe. They bequeathed us also their delusions which long served the good purpose of saving us from falling into greater ones. They left us the story of their errors and efforts, their triumphs and failures, their pains and joys, their loves and hates,—for warning or example. They expected our sympathy, because they toiled with the kindest wishes and hopes for us, and because they made our world. They cleared the land; they extirpated monsters; they tamed and taught the animals most useful to us. "*The mother of Kullervo awoke within her tomb, and from the deeps of the dust she cried to him, —'I have left thee the Dog, tied to a tree, that thou mayest go with him to the chase.'*(1)" They domesticated likewise the useful trees and plants; and they discovered the places and the powers of the metals. Later they created all that we call civilization,—trusting us to correct such mistakes as they could not help making. The sum of their toil is incalculable; and all that they have given us ought surely to be very sacred, very precious, if only by reason of the infinite pain and thought which it cost. Yet what Occidental dreams of saying daily, like the Shinto believer: —"*Ye forefathers of the generations, and of our families, and of our kindred,—unto you, the founders of our homes, we utter the gladness of our thanks*"?

None. It is not only because we think the dead cannot hear, but because we have not been trained for generations to exercise our powers of sympathetic mental representation except within a very narrow circle,—the family circle. The Occidental family circle is a very small affair indeed compared with the Oriental family circle. In this nineteenth century the Occidental family is almost disintegrated;—it practically means little more than husband, wife, and children well under age. The Oriental family means not only parents and their blood-kindred, but grandparents and their kindred, and great-grandparents, and all the dead behind them, This idea of the family cultivates sympathetic representation to such a degree that the range of the emotion belonging to such representation may extend, as in Japan, to many groups and sub-groups of living families, and even, in time of national peril, to the whole nation as one great family: a feeling much deeper than what we call patriotism. As a religious emotion the feeling is infinitely extended to all the past; the blended sense of love, of loyalty, and of gratitude is not less real, though necessarily more vague, than the feeling to living kindred.

In the West, after the destruction of antique society, no such feeling could remain. The beliefs that condemned the ancients to hell, and forbade the praise of their works,—the doctrine that trained us to return thanks for everything to the God of the Hebrews,—created habits of thought and habits of thoughtlessness, both inimical to every feeling of gratitude to the past. Then, with the decay of theology and the dawn of larger knowledge, came the teaching that the dead had no choice in their work,—they had obeyed necessity, and we had only received from them of necessity the results of necessity. And to-day we still fail to recognize that the necessity itself ought to compel our sympathies with those who obeyed it, and that its bequeathed results are as pathetic as they are precious. Such thoughts rarely occur to us even in regard to the work of the living who serve us. We consider the cost of a thing purchased or obtained to ourselves;—about its cost in effort to the producer we do not allow ourselves to think: indeed, we should be laughed at for any exhibition of conscience on the subject. And our equal insensibility to the pathetic meaning of the work of the past, and to that of the work of the present, largely explains the wastefulness of our civilization,—the reckless consumption by luxury of the labor of years in the pleasure of an hour,—the inhumanity of the thousands of unthinking rich, each of whom dissipates yearly in the gratification of totally unnecessary wants the price of a hundred human lives. The cannibals of civilization are unconsciously more cruel than those of savagery, and require much more flesh. The deeper humanity,—the cosmic emotion of humanity,—is essentially the enemy of useless luxury, and essentially opposed to any form of society which places no restraints upon the gratifications of sense or the pleasures of egotism.

In the Far East, on the other hand, the moral duty of simplicity of life has been taught from very ancient times, because ancestor-worship had developed and cultivated this cosmic emotion of humanity which we lack, but which we shall certainly be obliged to acquire at a later day, simply to save our selves from extermination, Two sayings of Iyeyasu exemplify the Oriental sentiment. When virtually master of the empire, this greatest of Japanese soldiers and statesmen was seen one day cleaning and smoothing with his own hands an old dusty pair of silk hakama or trousers. "What you see me do," he said to a retainer, "I am not doing because I think of the worth of the garment in itself, but because I think of what it needed to produce it. It is the result of the toil of a poor woman; and that is why I value it. *If we do not think, while using things, of the time and effort required to make them,—then our want of consideration puts us on a level with the beasts.*" Again, in the days of his greatest wealth, we hear of him rebuking his wife for wishing to furnish him too often with new clothing. "When I think," he protested, "of the multitudes around me, and of the generations to come after me, I feel it my duty to be very sparing, for their sake, of the goods in my possession." Nor has this spirit of simplicity yet departed from Japan. Even the Emperor and Empress, in the privacy of their own apartments, continue to live as simply as their subjects, and devote most of their revenue to the alleviation of public distress.

(1) Kalevala; thirty-sixth Rune.

V

It is through the teachings of evolution that there will ultimately be developed in the West a moral recognition of duty to the past like that which ancestor-worship created in the Far East. For even to-day whoever has mastered the first principles of the new philosophy cannot look at the commonest product of man's handiwork without perceiving something of its evolutional history. The most ordinary utensil will appear to him not the mere product of individual capacity on the part of carpenter or potter, smith or cutler, but the product of experiment continued through thousands of years with methods, with materials, and with forms. Nor will it be possible for him to consider the vast time and toil necessitated in the evolution, of any mechanical appliance, and yet experience no generous sentiment. Coming generations must think of the material bequests of the past in relation to dead humanity.

But in the development of this "cosmic emotion" of humanity, a much more powerful factor than recognition of our material indebtedness to the past will be the recognition of our psychical indebtedness. For we owe to the dead our immaterial world also,—the world that lives within us,—the world of all that is lovable in impulse, emotion, thought. Whosoever understands scientifically what human goodness is, and the terrible cost of making it, can find in the commonest phases of the humblest lives that beauty, which is divine, and can feel that in one sense our dead are truly gods.

So long as we supposed the woman soul one in itself,—a something specially created to fit one particular physical being,—the beauty and the wonder of mother-love could never be fully revealed to us. But with deeper knowledge we must perceive that the inherited love of myriads of millions of dead mothers has been treasured up in one life;—that only thus can be interpreted the infinite sweetness of the speech which the infant hears,—the infinite tenderness of the look of caress which meets its gaze. Unhappy the mortal who has not known these; yet what mortal can adequately speak of them! Truly is mother-love divine; for everything by human recognition called divine is summed up in that love; and every woman uttering and transmitting its highest expression is more than the mother of man: she is the *Mater Dei*.

Needless to speak here about the ghostliness of first love, sexual love, which is illusion,—because the passion and the beauty of the dead revive in it, to dazzle, to delude; and to bewitch. It is very, very wonderful; but it is not all good, because it is not all true. The real charm of woman in herself is that which comes later,—when all the illusions fade away to reveal a reality, lovelier than any illusion, which has been evolving behind the phantom-curtain of them. What is the divine magic of the woman thus perceived? Only the affection, the sweetness, the faith, the unselfishness, the intuitions of millions of buried hearts. All live again;—all throb anew, in every fresh warm beat of her own.

Certain amazing faculties exhibited in the highest social life tell in another way the story of soul structure built up by dead lives. Wonderful is the man who can really "be all things to all men," or the woman who can make herself twenty, fifty, a hundred different women,—comprehending all, penetrating all, unerring to estimate all others;—seeming to have no individual self, but only selves innumerable;—able to meet each varying personality with a soul exactly toned to the tone of that to be encountered. Rare these characters are, but not so rare that the traveler is unlikely to meet one or two of them in any cultivated society which he has a chance of studying. They are essentially multiple beings,—so visibly multiple that even those who think of the Ego as single have to describe them as "highly complex." Nevertheless this manifestation of forty or fifty different characters in the same person is a phenomenon so remarkable (especially remarkable because it is commonly manifested in youth long before relative experience could possibly account for it) that I cannot but wonder how few persons frankly realize its signification.

So likewise with what have been termed the "intuitions" of some forms of genius,—particularly those which relate to the representation of the emotions. A Shakespeare would always remain incomprehensible on the ancient soul-theory. Taine attempted to explain him by the phrase, "a perfect imagination;"—and the phrase reaches far in the truth. But what is the meaning of a perfect imagination? Enormous multiplicity of soul-life,—countless past existences revived in one. Nothing else can explain it…. It is not however, in the world of pure intellect that the story of psychical complexity is most admirable: it is in the world which speaks to our simplest emotions of love honor, sympathy, heroism.

"But by such a theory," some critic may observe, "the source of impulses to heroism is also the source of the impulses that people jails. Both are of the dead." This is true. We inherited evil as well as good. Being composites only,—still evolving, still becoming,—we inherit imperfections. But the survival of the fittest in impulses is certainly proven by the average moral condition of humanity,—using the word "fittest" in its ethical sense. In spite of all the misery and vice and crime, nowhere so terribly developed as under our own so-called Christian civilization, the fact must be patent to any one who has lived much, traveled much, and thought much, that the mass of humanity is good, and therefore that the vast majority of impulses bequeathed us by past humanity is good. Also it is certain that the more normal a social condition, the better its humanity. Through all the past the good Kami have always managed to keep the bad Kami from controlling the world. And with the acceptation of this truth, our future ideas of wrong and of right must take immense expansion. Just as a heroism, or any act of pure goodness for a noble end, must assume a preciousness heretofore unsuspected,—so a real crime must come to be regarded as a crime less against the existing individual or society, than against the sum of human experience, and the whole past struggle of ethical aspiration. Real goodness will, therefore, be more prized, and real crime less leniently judged. And the early Shinto teaching, that no code of ethics is necessary,—that the right rule of human conduct can always be known by consulting the heart,—is a teaching which will doubtless be accepted by a more perfect humanity than that of the present.

VI

"Evolution" the reader may say, "does indeed show through its doctrine of heredity that the living are in one sense really controlled by the dead. But it also shows that the dead are within us, not without us. They are part of us;—there is no proof that they have any existence which is not our own. Gratitude to the past would, therefore, be gratitude to ourselves; love of the dead would be self-love. So that your attempt at analogy ends in the absurd."

No. Ancestor-worship in its primitive form may be a symbol only of truth. It may be an index or foreshadowing only of the new moral duty which larger knowledge must force upon as the duty of reverence and obedience to the sacrificial past of human ethical experience. But it may also be much more. The facts of heredity can never afford but half an explanation of the facts of psychology. A plant produces ten, twenty, a hundred plants without yielding up its own life in the process. An animal gives birth to many young, yet lives on with all its physical capacities and its small powers of thought undiminished. Children are born; and the parents survive them. Inherited the mental life certainly is, not less than the physical; yet the reproductive cells, the least specialized of all cells, whether in plant or in animal, never take away, but only repeat the parental being. Continually multiplying, each conveys and transmits the whole experience of a race; yet leaves the whole experience of the race behind it. Here is the marvel inexplicable: the self-multiplication of physical and psychical being,—life after life thrown off from the parent life, each to become complete and reproductive. Were all the parental life given to the offspring, heredity might be said to favor the doctrine of materialism. But like the deities of Hindoo legend, the Self multiplies and still remains the same, with full capacities for continued multiplication. Shinto has its doctrine of souls multiplying by fission; but the facts of psychological emanation are infinitely more wonderful than any theory.

The great religions have recognized that heredity could not explain the whole question of self,—could not account for the fate of the original residual self. So they have generally united in holding the inner independent of the outer being. Science can no more fully decide the issues they have raised than it can decide the nature of Reality-in-itself. Again we may vainly ask, What becomes of the forces which constituted the vitality of a dead plant? Much more difficult the question, What becomes of the sensations which formed the psychical life of a dead man?—since nobody can explain the simplest sensation. We know only that during life certain active forces within the body of the plant or the body of the man adjusted themselves continually to outer forces; and that after the interior forces could no longer respond to the pressure of the exterior forces,—then the body in which the former were stored was dissolved into the elements out of which it had been built up. We know nothing more of the ultimate nature of those elements than we know of the ultimate nature of the tendencies which united them. But we have more right to believe the ultimates of life persist after the dissolution of the forms they created, than to believe they cease. The theory of spontaneous generation (misnamed, for only in a qualified sense can the term "spontaneous" be applied to the theory of the beginnings of mundane life) is a theory which the evolutionist must accept, and which can frighten none aware of the evidence of chemistry that matter itself is in evolution. The real theory (not the theory of organized life beginning in bottled infusions, but of the life primordial arising upon a planetary surface) has enormous—nay, infinite—spiritual significance. It requires the belief that all potentialities of life and thought and emotion pass from nebula to universe, from system to system, from star to planet or moon, and again back to cyclonic storms of atomicity; it means that tendencies survive sunburnings,—survive all cosmic evolutions and disintegrations. The elements are evolutionary products only; and the difference of universe from universe must be the creation of tendencies,—of a form of heredity too vast and complex for imagination. There is no chance. There is only law. Each fresh evolution must be influenced by previous evolutions,—just as each individual human life is influenced by the experience of all the lives in its ancestral chain. Must not the tendencies even of the ancestral forms of matter be inherited by the forms of matter to come; and may not the acts and thoughts of men even now be helping to shape the character of future worlds? No longer is it possible to say that the dreams of the Alchemists were absurdities. And no longer can we even assert that all material phenomena are not determined, as in the thought of the ancient East, by soul-polarities.

Whether our dead do or do not continue to dwell without us as well as within us,—a question not to be decided in our present undeveloped state of comparative blindness,—certain it is that the testimony of cosmic facts accords with one weird belief of Shinto: the belief that all things are determined by the dead,—whether by ghosts of men or ghosts of worlds. Even as our personal lives are ruled by the now viewless lives of the past, so doubtless the life of our Earth, and of the system to which it belongs, is ruled by ghosts of spheres innumerable: dead universes,—dead suns and planets and moons,—as forms long since dissolved into the night, but as forces immortal and eternally working.

Back to the Sun, indeed, like the Shintoist, we can trace our descent; yet we know that even there the beginning of us was not. Infinitely more remote in time than a million sun-lives was that beginning,—if it can truly be said there was a beginning. The teaching of Evolution is that we are one with that unknown Ultimate, of which matter and human mind are but ever-changing manifestations. The teaching of Evolution is also that each of us is many, yet that all of us are still one with each other and with the cosmos;—that we must know all past humanity not only in ourselves, but likewise in the preciousness and beauty of every fellow-life;—that we can best love ourselves in others;—that we shall best serve ourselves in others;—that forms are but veils and phantoms;—and that to the formless Infinite alone really belong all human emotions, whether of the living or the dead.

XV

KIMIKO

Wasuraruru
Mi naran to omo
Kokoro koso
Wasure nu yori mo
Omoi nari-kere.

"To wish to be forgotten by the beloved is a soul-task harder far than trying not to forget."—Poem by Kimiko.

I

The name is on a paper-lantern at the entrance of a house in the Street of the Geisha.

Seen at night the street is one of the queerest in the world. It is narrow as a gangway; and the dark shining woodwork of the house-fronts, all tightly closed,—each having a tiny sliding door with paper-panes that look just like frosted glass,—makes you think of first-class passenger-cabins. Really the buildings are several stories high; but you do not observe this at once,—especially if there be no moon,—because only the lower stories are illuminated up to their awnings, above which all is darkness. The illumination is made by lamps behind the narrow paper-paned doors, and by the paper-lanterns hanging outside,—one at every door. You look down the street between two lines of these lanterns,—lines converging far-off into one motionless bar of yellow light. Some of the lanterns are egg-shaped, some cylindrical; others four-sided or six-sided; and Japanese characters are beautifully written upon them. The street is very quiet,—silent as a display of cabinet-work in some great exhibition after closing-time. This is because the inmates are mostly away,—at tending banquets and other festivities. Their life is of the night.

The legend upon the first lantern to the left as you go south is "Kinoya: uchi O-Kata;" and that means The House of Gold wherein O-Kata dwells. The lantern to the right tells of the House of Nishimura, and of a girl Miyotsuru,—which name signifies The Stork Magnificently Existing. Next upon the left comes the House of Kajita;—and in that house are Kohana, the Flower-Bud, and Hinako, whose face is pretty as the face of a doll. Opposite is the House Nagaye, wherein live Kimika and Kimiko.... And this luminous double litany of names is half-a-mile long.

The inscription on the lantern of the last-named house reveals the relationship between Kimika and Kimiko,—and yet something more; for Kimiko is styled Ni-dai-me, an honorary untranslatable title which signifies that she is only Kimiko No.2. Kimika is the teacher and mistress: she has educated two geisha, both named, or rather renamed by her, Kimiko; and this use of the same name twice is proof positive that the first Kimiko—Ichi-dai-me—must have been celebrated. The professional appellation borne by an unlucky or unsuccessful geisha is never given to her successor. If you should ever have good and sufficient reason to enter the house,—pushing open that lantern-slide of a door which sets a gong-bell ringing to announce visits,—you might be able to see Kimika, provided her little troupe be not engaged for the evening. You would find her a very intelligent person, and well worth talking to. She can tell, when she pleases, the most remarkable stories,—real flesh-and-blood stories,—true stories of human nature. For the Street of the Geisha is full of traditions,—tragic, comic, melodramatic;—every house has its memories;—and Kimika knows them all. Some are very, very terrible; and some would make you laugh; and some would make you think. The story of the first Kimiko belongs to the last class. It is not one of the most extraordinary; but it is one of the least difficult for Western people to understand.

II

There is no more Ichi-dai-me Kimiko: she is only a remembrance. Kimika was quite young when she called that Kimiko her professional sister.

"An exceedingly wonderful girl," is what Kimika says of Kimiko. To win any renown in her profession, a geisha must be pretty or very clever; and the famous ones are usually both,—having been selected at a very early age by their trainers according to the promise of such qualities, even the commoner class of singing-girls must have some charm in their best years, —if only that *beaute du diable* which inspired the Japanese proverb that even a devil is pretty at eighteen(1). But Kimiko was much more than pretty. She was according to the Japanese ideal of beauty; and that standard is not reached by one woman in a hundred thousand. Also she was more than clever: she was accomplished. She composed very dainty poems,— could arrange flowers exquisitely, perform tea-ceremonies faultlessly, embroider, make silk mosaic: in short, she was genteel. And her first public appearance made a flutter in the fast world of Kyoto. It was evident that she could make almost any conquest she pleased, and that fortune was before her.

But it soon became evident, also, that she had been perfectly trained for her profession. She had been taught how to conduct herself under almost any possible circumstances; for what she could not have known Kimika knew everything about: the power of beauty, and the weakness of passion; the craft of promises and the worth of indifference; and all the folly and evil in the hearts of men. So Kimiko made few mistakes and shed few tears. By and by she proved to be, as Kimika wished,—slightly dangerous. So a lamp is to night-fliers: otherwise some of them would put it out. The duty of the lamp is to make pleasant things visible: it has no malice. Kimiko had no malice, and was not too dangerous. Anxious parents discovered that she did not want to enter into respectable families, nor even to lend herself to any serious romances. But she was not particularly merciful to that class of youths who sign documents with their own blood, and ask a dancing-girl to cut off the extreme end of the little finger of her left hand as a pledge of eternal affection. She was mischievous enough with them to cure them of their folly. Some rich folks who offered her lands and houses on condition of owning her, body and soul, found her less merciful. One proved generous enough to purchase her freedom unconditionally, at a price which made Kimika a rich woman; and Kimiko was grateful,—but she remained a geisha. She managed her rebuffs with too much tact to excite hate, and knew how to heal despairs in most cases. There were exceptions, of course. One old man, who thought life not worth living unless he could get Kimiko all to himself, invited her to a banquet one evening, and asked her to drink wine with him. But Kimika, accustomed to read faces, deftly substituted tea (which has precisely the same color) for Kimiko's wine, and so instinctively saved the girl's precious life,—for only ten minutes later the soul of the silly host was on its way to the Meido alone, and doubtless greatly disappointed…. After that night Kimika watched over Kimiko as a wild cat guards her kitten.

The kitten became a fashionable mania, a craze,—a delirium,—one of the great sights and sensations of the period. There is a foreign prince who remembers her name: he sent her a gift of diamonds which she never wore. Other presents in multitude she received from all who could afford the luxury of pleasing her; and to be in her good graces, even for a day, was the ambition of the "gilded youth." Nevertheless she allowed no one to imagine himself a special favorite, and refused to make any contracts for perpetual affection. To any protests on the subject she answered that she knew her place. Even respectable women spoke not unkindly of her,—because her name never figured in any story of family unhappiness. She really kept her place. Time seemed to make her more charming. Other geisha grew into fame, but no one was even classed with her. Some manufacturers secured the sole right to use her photograph for a label; and that label made a fortune for the firm.

But one day the startling news was abroad that Kimiko had at last shown a very soft heart. She had actually said good-by to Kimika, and had gone away with somebody able to give her all the pretty dresses she could wish for,—somebody eager to give her social position also, and to silence gossip about her naughty past,—somebody willing to die for her ten times over, and already half-dead for love of her. Kimika said that a fool had tried to kill himself because of Kimiko, and that Kimiko had taken pity on him, and nursed him back to foolishness. Taiko Hideyoshi had said that there were only two things in this world which he feared,—a fool and a dark night. Kimika had always been afraid of a fool; and a fool had taken Kimiko away. And she added, with not unselfish tears, that Kimiko would never come back to her: it was a case of love on both sides for the time of several existences.

Nevertheless, Kimika was only half right. She was very shrewd indeed; but she had never been able to see into certain private chambers in the soul of Kimiko. If she could have seen, she would have screamed for astonishment.

(1) Oni mo jiuhachi, azami no hana. There is a similar saying of a dragon: ja mo hatachi ("even a dragon at twenty").

III

Between Kimiko and other geisha there was a difference of gentle blood. Before she took a professional name, her name was Ai, which, written with the proper character, means love. Written with another character the same word-sound signifies grief. The story of Ai was a story of both grief and love.

She had been nicely brought up. As a child she had been sent to a private school kept by an old samurai,—where the little girls squatted on cushions before little writing-tables twelve inches high, and where the teachers taught without salary. In these days when teachers get better salaries than civil-service officials, the teaching is not nearly so honest or so pleasant as it used to be. A servant always accompanied the child to and from the school-house, carrying her books, her writing-box, her kneeling cushion, and her little table.

Afterwards she attended an elementary public school. The first "modern" text-books had just been issued,—containing Japanese translations of English, German, and French stories about honor and duty and heroism, excellently chosen, and illustrated with tiny innocent pictures of Western people in costumes never of this world. Those dear pathetic little text-books are now curiosities: they have long been superseded by pretentious compilations much less lovingly and sensibly edited. Ai learned well. Once a year, at examination time, a great official would visit the school, and talk to the children as if they were all his own, and stroke each silky head as he distributed the prizes. He is now a retired statesman, and has doubtless forgotten Ai;—and in the schools of to-day nobody caresses little girls, or gives them prizes.

Then came those reconstructive changes by which families of rank were reduced to obscurity and poverty; and Ai had to leave school. Many great sorrows followed, till there remained to her only her mother and an infant sister. The mother and Ai could do little but weave; and by weaving alone they could not earn enough to live. House and lands first,—then, article by article, all things not necessary to existence—heirlooms, trinkets, costly robes, crested lacquer-ware—passed cheaply to those whom misery makes rich, and whose wealth is called by the people *Namida no kane*,—"the Money of Tears." Help from the living was scanty,—for most of the samurai-families of kin were in like distress. But when there was nothing left to sell,—not even Ai's little school-books,—help was sought from the dead.

For it was remembered that the father of Ai's father had been buried with his sword, the gift of a daimyo; and that the mountings of the weapon were of gold. So the grave was opened, and the grand hilt of curious workmanship exchanged for a common one, and the ornaments of the lacquered sheath removed. But the good blade was not taken, because the warrior might need it. Ai saw his face as he sat erect in the great red-clay urn which served in lieu of coffin to the samurai of high rank when buried by the ancient rite. His features were still recognizable after all those years of sepulture; and he seemed to nod a grim assent to what had been done as his sword was given back to him.

At last the mother of Ai became too weak and ill to work at the loom; and the gold of the dead had been spent. Ai said:—"Mother, I know there is but one thing now to do. Let me be sold to the dancing-girls." The mother wept, and made no reply. Ai did not weep, but went out alone.

She remembered that in other days, when banquets were given in her father's house, and dancers served the wine, a free geisha named Kimika had often caressed her. She went straight to the house of Kimika. "I want you to buy me," said Ai;—"and I want a great deal of money." Kimika laughed, and petted her, and made her eat, and heard her story,—which was bravely told, without one tear. "My child," said Kimika, "I cannot give you a great deal of money; for I have very little. But this I can do:—I can promise to support your mother. That will be better than to give her much money for you,—because your mother, my child, has been a great lady, and therefore cannot know how to use money cunningly. Ask your honored mother to sign the bond,—promising that you will stay with me till you are twenty-four years old, or until such time as you can pay me back. And what money I can now spare, take home with you as a free gift."

Thus Ai became a geisha; and Kimika renamed her Kimiko, and kept the pledge to maintain the mother and the child-sister. The mother died before Kimiko became famous; the little sister was put to school. Afterwards those things already told came to pass.

The young man who had wanted to die for love of a dancing-girl was worthy of better things. He was an only son and his parents, wealthy and titled people, were willing to make any sacrifice for him,—even that of accepting a geisha for daughter-in-law. Moreover they were not altogether displeased with Kimiko, because of her sympathy for their boy.

Before going away, Kimiko attended the wedding of her young sister, Ume, who had just finished school. She was good and pretty. Kimiko had made the match, and used her wicked knowledge of men in making it. She chose a very plain, honest, old-fashioned merchant,—a man who could not have been bad, even if he tried. Ume did not question the wisdom of her sister's choice, which time proved fortunate.

IV

It was in the period of the fourth moon that Kimiko was carried away to the home prepared for her,—a place in which to forget all the unpleasant realities of life,—a sort of fairy-palace lost in the charmed repose of great shadowy silent high-walled gardens. Therein she might have felt as one reborn, by reason of good deeds, into the realm of Horai. But the spring passed, and the summer came,—and Kimiko remained simply Kimiko. Three times she had contrived, for reasons unspoken, to put off the wedding-day.

In the period of the eighth moon, Kimiko ceased to be playful, and told her reasons very gently but very firmly:—"It is time that I should say what I have long delayed saying. For the sake of the mother who gave me life, and for the sake of my little sister, I have lived in hell. All that is past; but the scorch of the fire is upon me, and there is no power that can take it away. It is not for such as I to enter into an honored family,—nor to bear you a son, —nor to build up your house…. Suffer me to speak; for in the knowing of wrong I am very, very much wiser than you…. Never shall I be your wife to become your shame. I am your companion only, your play-fellow, your guest of an hour, —and this not for any gifts. When I shall be no longer with you nay! certainly that day must come!—you will have clearer sight. I shall still be dear to you, but not in the same way as now—which is foolishness. You will remember these words out of my heart. Some true sweet lady will be chosen for you, to become the mother of your children. I shall see them; but the place of a wife I shall never take, and the joy of a mother I must never know. I am only your folly, my beloved,—an illusion, a dream, a shadow flitting across your life. Somewhat more in later time I may become, but a wife to you never, neither in this existence nor in the next. Ask me again-and I go."

In the period of the tenth moon, and without any reason imaginable, Kimiko disappeared,—vanished,—utterly ceased to exist.

V

Nobody knew when or how or whither she had gone. Even in the neighborhood of the home she had left, none had seen her pass. At first it seemed that she must soon return. Of all her beautiful and precious things- her robes, her ornaments, her presents: a fortune in themselves—she had taken nothing. But weeks passed without word or sign; and it was feared that something terrible had befallen her. Rivers were dragged, and wells were searched. Inquiries were made by telegraph and by letter. Trusted servants were sent to look for her. Rewards were offered for any news—especially a reward to Kimika, who was really attached to the girl, and would have been only too happy to find her without any reward at all. But the mystery remained a mystery. Application to the authorities would have been useless: the fugitive had done no wrong, broken no law; and the vast machinery of the imperial police-system was not to be set in motion by the passionate whim of a boy. Months grew into years; but neither Kimika, nor the little sister in Kyoto, nor any one of the thousands who had known and admired the beautiful dancer, ever saw Kimiko again.

But what she had foretold came true;—for time dries all tears and quiets all longing; and even in Japan one does not really try to die twice for the same despair. The lover of Kimiko became wiser; and there was found for him a very sweet person for wife, who gave him a son. And other years passed; and there was happiness in the fairy-home where Kimiko had once been.

There came to that home one morning, as if seeking alms, a traveling nun; and the child, hearing her Buddhist cry of "*Ha—i! ha—i!*" ran to the gate. And presently a house-servant, bringing out the customary gift of rice, wondered to see the nun caressing the child, and whispering to him. Then the little one cried to the servant, "Let me give!"—and the nun pleaded from under the veiling shadow of her great straw hat: "Honorably allow the child to give me." So the boy put the rice into the mendicant's bowl. Then she thanked him, and asked:—"Now will you say again for me the little word which I prayed you to tell your honored father?" And the child lisped: —"*Father, one whom you will never see again in this world, says that her heart is glad because she has seen your son.*"

The nun laughed softly, and caressed him again, and passed away swiftly; and the servant wondered more than ever, while the child ran to tell his father the words of the mendicant.

But the father's eyes dimmed as he heard the words, and he wept over his boy. For he, and only he, knew who had been at the gate, —and the sacrificial meaning of all that had been hidden.

Now he thinks much, but tells his thought to no one.

He knows that the space between sun and sun is less than the space between himself and the woman who loved him.

He knows it were vain to ask in what remote city, in what fantastic riddle of narrow nameless streets, in what obscure little temple known only to the poorest poor, she waits for the darkness before the Dawn of the Immeasurable Light,—when the Face of the Teacher will smile upon her,—when the Voice of the Teacher will say to her, in tones of sweetness deeper than ever came from human lover's lips:—"*O my daughter in the Law, thou hast practiced the perfect way; thou hast believed and understood the highest truth;—therefore come I now to meet and to welcome thee!*"

APPENDIX

THREE POPULAR BALLADS

Read before the Asiatic Society of Japan, October 17, 1894.

During the spring of 1891, I visited the settlement in Matsue, Izumo, of an outcast people known as the *yama-no-mono*. Some results of the visit were subsequently communicated to the "Japan Mail," in a letter published June 13, 1891, and some extracts from that letter I think it may be worth while to cite here, by way of introduction to the subject of the present paper.

"The settlement is at the southern end of Matsue in a tiny valley, or rather hollow among the hills which form a half-circle behind the city. Few Japanese of the better classes have ever visited such a village; and even the poorest of the common people shun the place as they would shun a centre of contagion; for the idea of defilement, both moral and physical, is still attached to the very name of its inhabitants. Thus, although the settlement is within half an hour's walk from the heart of the city, probably not half a dozen of the thirty-six thousand residents of Matsue have visited it.

"There are four distinct outcast classes in Matsue and its environs: the *hachiya*, the *koya-no-mono*, the *yama-no-mono*, and the *eta* of Suguta.

"There are two settlements of *hachiya*. These were formerly the public executioners, and served under the police in various capacities. Although by ancient law the lowest class of pariahs, their intelligence was sufficiently cultivated by police service and by contact with superiors to elevate them in popular opinion above the other outcasts. They are now manufacturers of bamboo cages and baskets. They are said to be descendants of the family and retainers of Taira-no-Masakado-Heishino, the only man in Japan who ever seriously conspired to seize the imperial thrones by armed force, and who was killed by the famous general Taira-no-Sadamori.

"The *koya-no-mono* are slaughterers and dealers in hides. They are never allowed to enter any house in Matsue except the shop of a dealer in geta and other footgear. Originally vagrants, they were permanently settled in Matsue by some famous daimyo, who built for them small houses—*koya*—on the bank of the canal. Hence their name. As for the *eta* proper, their condition and calling are too familiar to need comment in this connection.

"The *yama-no-mono* are so called because they live among the hills (*yama*) at the southern end of Matsue. They have a monopoly of the rag-and-waste-paper business, and are buyers of all sorts of refuse, from old bottles to broken-down machinery. Some of them are rich. Indeed, the whole class is, compared with other outcast classes, prosperous. Nevertheless, public prejudice against them is still almost as strong as in the years previous to the abrogation of the special laws concerning them. Under no conceivable circumstances could any of them obtain employment as servants. Their prettiest girls in old times often became *joro*; but at no time could they enter a *joroya* in any neighboring city, much less in their own, so they were sold to establishments in remote places. A *yama-no-mono* to-day could not even become a *kurumaya*. He could not obtain employment as a common laborer in any capacity, except by going to some distant city where he could hope to conceal his origin. But if detected under such conditions he would run serious risk of being killed by his fellow-laborers. Under any circumstance it would be difficult for a *yama-no-mono* to pass himself off for a *heimin*. Centuries of isolation and prejudice have fixed and moulded the manners of the class in recognizable ways; and even its language has become a special and curious dialect.

"I was anxious to see something of a class so singularly situated and specialized; and I had the good fortune to meet a Japanese gentleman who, although belonging to the highest class of Matsue, was kind enough to agree to accompany me to their village, where he had never been himself. On the way thither he told me many curious things about the *yama-no-mono*. In feudal times these people had been kindly treated by the samurai; and they were often allowed or invited to enter the courts of samurai dwellings to sing and dance, for which performances they were paid. The songs and the dances with which they were able to entertain even those aristocratic families were known to no other people, and were called Daikoku-mai. Singing the Daikoku-mai was, in fact, the special hereditary art of the *yama-no-mono*, and represented their highest comprehension of aesthetic and emotional matters. In former times they could not obtain admittance to a respectable theatre; and, like the *hachiya*, had theatres of their own. It would be interesting, my friend added, to learn the origin of their songs and their dances; for their songs are not in their own special dialect, but in pure Japanese. And that they should have been able to preserve this oral literature without deterioration is especially remarkable from the fact that the *yama-no-mono* were never taught to read or write. They could not even avail themselves of those new educational opportunities which the era of Meiji has given to the masses; prejudice is still far too strong to allow of their children being happy in a public school. A small special school might be possible, though there would perhaps be no small difficulty in obtaining willing teachers(1).

"The hollow in which the village stands is immediately behind the Buddhist cemetery of Tokoji. The settlement has its own Shinto temple. I was extremely surprised at the aspect of the place; for I had expected to see a good deal of ugliness and filth. On the contrary, I saw a multitude of neat dwellings, with pretty gardens about them, and pictures on the walls of the rooms. There were many trees; the village was green with shrubs and plants, and picturesque to an extreme degree; for, owing to the irregularity of the ground, the tiny streets climbed up and down hill at all sorts of angles,—the loftiest street being fifty or sixty feet above the lowermost. A large public bath-house and a public laundry bore evidence that the *yama-no-mono* liked clean linen as well as their *heimin* neighbors on the other side of the hill.

"A crowd soon gathered to look at the strangers who had come to their village,—a rare event for them. The faces I saw seemed much like the faces of the *heimin*, except that I fancied the ugly ones were uglier, making the pretty ones appear more pretty by contrast. There were one or two sinister faces, recalling faces of gypsies that I had seen; while some little girls, on the other hand, had remarkably pleasing features. There were no exchanges of civilities, as upon meeting *heimin*; a Japanese of the better class would as soon think of taking off his hat to a *yama-no-mono* as a West-Indian planter would think of bowing to a negro. The *yama-no-mono* themselves usually show by their attitude that they expect no forms. None of the men saluted us; but some of the women, on being kindly addressed, made obeisance. Other women, weaving coarse straw sandals (an inferior quality of zori), would answer only 'yes' or 'no' to questions, and seemed to be suspicious of us. My friend called my attention to the fact that the women were dressed differently from Japanese women of the ordinary classes. For example, even among the very poorest *heimin* there are certain accepted laws of costume; there are certain colors which may or may not be worn, according to age. But even elderly women among these people wear obi of bright red or variegated hues, and kimono of a showy tint.

"Those of the women seen in the city street, selling or buying, are the elders only. The younger stay at home. The elderly women always go into town with large baskets of a peculiar shape, by which the fact that they are *yama-no-mono* is at once known. Numbers of these baskets were visible, principally at the doors of the smaller dwellings. They are carried on the back, and are used to contain all that the *yama-no-mono* buy,—old paper, old wearing apparel, bottles, broken glass, and scrap-metal.

"A woman at last ventured to invite us to her house, to look at some old colored prints she wished to sell. Thither we went, and were as nicely received as in a *heimin* residence. The pictures —including a number of drawings by Hiroshige—proved to be worth buying; and my friend then asked if we could have the pleasure of hearing the Daikoku-mai. To my great satisfaction the proposal was well received; and on our agreeing to pay a trifle to each singer, a small band of neat-looking young girls, whom we had not seen before, made their appearance, and prepared to sing, while an old woman made ready to dance. Both the old woman and the girls provided themselves with curious instruments for the performance. Three girls had instruments shaped like mallets, made of paper and bamboo: these were intended to represent the hammer of Dai-koku(2); they were held in the left hand, a fan being waved in the right. Other girls were provided with a kind of castanets,—two flat pieces of hard dark wood, connected by a string. Six girls formed in a line before the house. The old woman took her place facing the girls, holding in her hands two little sticks, one stick being notched along a part of its length. By drawing it across the other stick, a curious rattling noise was made.

"My friend pointed out to me that the singers formed two distinct parties, of three each. Those bearing the hammer and fan were the Daikoku band: they were to sing the ballads. Those with the castanets were the Ebisu party and formed the chorus.

"The old woman rubbed her little sticks together, and from the throats of the Daikoku band there rang out a clear, sweet burst of song, quite different from anything I had heard before in Japan, while the tapping of the castanets kept exact time to the syllabification of the words, which were very rapidly uttered. When the first three girls had sung a certain number of lines, the voices of the other three joined in, producing a very pleasant though untrained harmony; and all sang the burden together. Then the Daikoku party began another verse; and, after a certain interval, the chorus was again sung. In the meanwhile the old woman was dancing a very fantastic dance which provoked laughter from the crowd, occasionally chanting a few comic words.

"The song was not comic, however; it was a very pathetic ballad entitled 'Yaoya O-Shichi.' Yaoya O-Shichi was a beautiful girl, who set fire to her own house in order to obtain another meeting with her lover, an acolyte in a temple where she expected that her family would be obliged to take refuge after the fire. But being detected and convicted of arson, she was condemned by the severe law of that age to be burnt alive. The sentence was carried into effect; but the youth and beauty of the victim, and the motive of her offense, evoked a sympathy in the popular heart which found later expression in song and, drama.

"None of the performers, except the old woman, lifted the feet from the ground while singing—but all swayed their bodies in time to the melody.

The singing lasted more than one hour, during which the voices never failed in their quality; and yet, so far from being weary of it, and although I could not understand a word uttered, I felt very sorry when it was all over. And with the pleasure received there came to the foreign listener also a strong sense of sympathy for the young singers, victims of a prejudice so ancient that its origin is no longer known."

(1) Since the time this letter to the Mail was written, a primary school has been established for the yama-no-mono, through the benevolence of Matsue citizens superior to prejudice. The undertaking did not escape severe local criticism, but it seems to have proved successful.

(2) Daikoku is the popular God of Wealth. Ebisu is the patron of labor. See, for the history of these deities, an article (translated) entitled "The Seven Gods of Happiness," by Carlo Puini, vol. iii. Transactions of the Asiatic Society. See, also, for an account of their place in Shinto worship, Glimpses of Unfamiliar Japan, vol. 1.

The foregoing extracts from my letter to the "Mail" tell the history of my interest in the Daikoku-mai. At a later time I was able to procure, through the kindness of my friend Nishida Sentaro, of Matsue, written copies of three of the ballads as sung by the *yama-no-mono*; and translations of these were afterwards made for me. I now venture to offer my prose renderings of the ballads,—based on the translations referred to,—as examples of folk-song not devoid of interest. An absolutely literal rendering, executed with the utmost care, and amply supplied with explanatory notes, would be, of course, more worthy the attention of a learned society. Such a version would, however, require a knowledge of Japanese which I do not possess, as well as much time and patient labor. Were the texts in themselves of value sufficient to justify a scholarly translation, I should not have attempted any translation at all; but I felt convinced that their interest was of a sort which could not be much diminished by a free and easy treatment. From any purely literary point of view, the texts are disappointing, exhibiting no great power of imagination, and nothing really worthy to be called poetical art. While reading such verses, we find ourselves very far away indeed from the veritable poetry of Japan,—from those compositions which, with a few chosen syllables only, can either create a perfect colored picture in the mind, or bestir the finest sensations of memory with marvelous penetrative delicacy. The Daikoku-mai are extremely crude; and their long popularity has been due, I fancy, rather to the very interesting manner of singing them than to any quality which could permit us to compare them with the old English ballads.

The legends upon which these chants were based still exist in many other forms, including dramatic compositions. I need scarcely refer to the vast number of artistic suggestions which they have given, but I may observe that their influence in this regard has not yet passed away. Only a few months ago, I saw a number of pretty cotton prints, fresh from the mill, picturing Oguri-Hangwan making the horse Onikage stand upon a chessboard. Whether the versions of the ballads I obtained in Izumo were composed there or elsewhere I am quite unable to say; but the stories of Shuntoku-maru, Oguri-Hangwan, and Yaoya O-Shichi are certainly well known in every part of Japan.

Together with these prose translations, I submit to the Society the original texts, to which are appended some notes of interest about the local customs connected with the singing of the Daikoku-mai, about the symbols used by the dancers, and about the comic phrases chanted at intervals during the performances,—phrases of which the coarse humor sometimes forbids any

The fact, however, that few of those peculiarities which give so strange a charm to the old peasant-chants are noticeable in the Izumo manner of singing the Daikoku-mai would perhaps indicate that the latter are comparatively modern.

THE BALLAD OF SHUNTOKU-MARU

Ara!—Joyfully young Daikoko and Ebisu enter dancing

Shall we tell a tale, or shall we utter felicitations? A tale: then of what is it best that we should tell? Since we are bidden to your august house to relate a story, we shall relate the story of Shuntoku.

Surely there once lived, in the Province of Kawachi, a very rich man called Nobuyoshi. And his eldest son was called Shuntoku-maru.

When Shuntoku-maru, that eldest son, was only three years old, his mother died. And when he was five years old, there was given to him a stepmother.

When he was seven years old, his stepmother gave birth to a son who was called Otowaka-maru. And the two brothers grew up together.

When Shuntoku became sixteen years old, he went to Kyoto, to the temple of Tenjin-Sama, to make offerings to the god.

There he saw a thousand people going to the temple, and a thousand returning, and a thousand remaining: there was a gathering of three thousand persons(1).

Through that multitude the youngest daughter of a rich man called Hagiyama was being carried to the temple in a kago(2). Shuntoku also was traveling in a kago; and the two kago moved side by side along the way.

Gazing on the girl, Shuntoku fell in love with her. And the two exchanged looks and letters of love.

All this was told to the stepmother of Shuntoku by a servant that was a flatterer.

Then the stepmother began to think that should the youth remain in his father's home, the store-houses east and west, and the granaries north and south, and the house that stood in the midst, could never belong to Otowaka-maru.

Therefore she devised an evil thing, and spoke to her husband, saying, "Sir, my lord, may I have your honored permission to be free for seven days from the duties of the household?"

Her husband answered, "Yes, surely; but what is it that you wish to do for seven days?" She said to him: "Before being wedded to my lord, I made a vow to the August Deity of Kiyomidzu; and now I desire to go to the temple to fulfill that vow."

Said the master: "That is well. But which of the man servants or maid servants would you wish to go with you?" Then she made reply: "Neither man servant nor maid servant do I require. I wish to go all alone."

And without paying heed to any advice about her journey, she departed from the house, and made great haste to Kyoto.

Reaching the quarter Sanjo in the city of Kyoto, she asked the way to the street Kajiyamachi, which is the Street of the Smiths. And finding it, she saw three smithies side by side.

Going to the middle one, she greeted the smith, and asked him: "Sir smith, can you make some fine small work in iron?" And he answered: "Ay, lady, that I can."

Then she said: "Make me, I pray you, nine and forty nails without heads." But he answered: "I am of the seventh generation of a family of smiths; yet never did I hear till now of nails without heads, and such an order I cannot take. It were better that you should ask elsewhere."

"Nay," said she, "since I came first to you, I do not want to go elsewhere. Make them for me, I pray, sir smith." He answered: "Of a truth, if I make such nails, I must be paid a thousand ryo(3)."

She replied to him: "If you make them all for me, I care nothing whether you desire one thousand or two thousand ryo. Make them, I beseech you, sir smith." So the smith could not well refuse to make the nails.

He arranged all things rightly to honor the God of the Bellows(4). Then taking up his first hammer, he recited the Kongo-Sutra(5); taking up his second, he recited the Kwannon-Sutra; taking up his third, he recited the Amida-Sutra,—because he feared those nails might be used for a wicked purpose.

Thus in sorrow he finished the nails. Then was the woman much pleased. And receiving the nails in her left hand, she paid the money to the smith with her right, and bade him farewell, and went upon her way.

When she was gone, then the smith thought: "Surely I have in gold koban(6) the sum of a thousand ryo. But this life of ours is only like the resting-place of a traveler journeying, and I must show to others some pity and kindness. To those who are cold I will give clothing, and to those who are hungry I will give food."

And by announcing his intention in writings(7) set up at the boundaries of provinces and at the limits of villages, he was able to show his benevolence to many people.

On her way the woman stopped at the house of a painter, and asked the painter to paint for her a picture.

And the painter questioned her, sayings "Shall I paint you the picture of a very old plum-tree, or of an ancient pine?"

She said to him; "No: I want neither the picture of an old plum-tree nor of an ancient pine. I want the picture of a boy of sixteen years, having a stature of five feet, and two moles upon his face."

"That," said the painter, "will be an easy thing to paint." And he made the picture in a very little time. It was much like Shuntoku-maru; and the woman rejoiced as she departed.

With that picture of Shuntoku she hastened to Kiyomidzu; and she pasted the picture upon one of the pillars in the rear of the temple.

And with forty-seven out of the forty-nine nails she nailed the picture to the pillar; and with the two remaining nails she nailed the eyes.

Then feeling assured that she had put a curse upon Shuntoku, that wicked woman went home. And she said humbly, "I have returned;" and she pretended to be faithful and true.

(1) These numbers simply indicate a great multitude in the language of the people; they have no exact significance.

(2) Kago, a kind of palanquin.

(3) The ancient ryo or tael had a value approximating that of the dollar of 100 sen.

(4) Fuigo Sama, deity of smiths.

(5) "Diamond Sutra."

(6) Koban, a gold coin. There were koban of a great many curious shapes and designs. The most common form was a flat or oval disk, stamped with Chinese characters. Some koban were fully five inches in length by four in width.

(7) Public announcements are usually written upon small wooden tablets attached to a post; and in the country such announcements are still set up just as suggested in the ballad.

Now three or four months after the stepmother of Shuntoku had thus invoked evil upon him he became very sick. Then that stepmother secretly rejoiced.

And she spoke cunningly to Nobuyoshi, her husband, saying: "Sir, my lord, this sickness of Shuntoku seems to be a very bad sickness; and it is difficult to keep one having such sickness in the house of a rich man."

Then Nobuyoshi was much surprised, and sorrowed greatly; but, thinking to himself that indeed it could not be helped, he called Shuntoku to him, and said:—

"Son, this sickness which you have seems to be leprosy; and one having such a sickness cannot continue to dwell in this house.

"It were best for you, therefore, to make a pilgrimage through all the provinces, in the hope that you may be healed by divine influence.

"And my storehouses and my granaries I will not give to Otowaka-maru, but only to you, Shuntoku; so you must come back to us."

Poor Shuntoku, not knowing how wicked his stepmother was, besought her in his sad condition, saying: "Dear mother, I have been told that I must go forth and wander as a pilgrim.

"But now I am blind, and I cannot travel without difficulty. I should be content with one meal a day in place of three, and glad for permission to live in a corner of some storeroom or outhouse; but I should like to remain somewhere near my home.

"Will you not please permit me to stay, if only for a little time? Honored mother, I beseech you, let me stay."

But she answered: "As this trouble which you now have is only the beginning of the bad disease, it is not possible for me to suffer you to stay. You must go away from the house at once."

Then Shuntoku was forced out of the house by the servants, and into the yard, sorrowing greatly.

And the wicked stepmother, following, cried out: "As your father has commanded, you must go away at once, Shuntoku."

Shuntoku answered: "See, I have not even a traveling-dress. A pilgrim's gown and leggings I ought to have, and a pilgrim's wallet for begging."

At hearing these words, the wicked stepmother was glad; and she at once gave him all that he required.

Shuntoku received the things, and thanked her, and made ready to depart, even in his piteous state.

He put on the gown and hung a wooden mamori (charm) upon his breast(1), and he suspended the wallet about his neck. He put on his straw sandals and fastened them tightly, and took a bamboo staff in his hand, and placed a hat of woven rushes upon his head.

And saying, "Farewell, father; farewell, mother," poor Shuntoku started on his journey.

Sorrowfully Nobuyoshi accompanied his son a part of the way, saying: "It cannot be helped, Shuntoku. But if, through the divine favor of those august deities to whom that charm is dedicated, your disease should become cured, then come back to us at once, my son."

Hearing from his father these kind words of farewell, Shuntoku felt much happier, and covering his face with the great rush hat, so as not to be known to the neighbors, he went on alone.

But in a little while, finding his limbs so weak that he was afraid he could not go far, and feeling his heart always drawn back toward his home, so that he could not help often stopping and turning his face thither, he became sad again.

(1) See Professor Chamberlain's "Notes on some Minor Japanese Religious Practices," for full details of pilgrimages and pilgrim costumes, in

Journal of the Anthropological Institute (1898). The paper is excellently illustrated.

Since it would have been difficult for him to enter any dwelling, he had often to sleep under pine-trees or in the forests; but sometimes he was lucky enough to find shelter in some wayside shrine containing images of the Buddhas.

And once in the darkness of the morning, before the breaking of the day, in the hour when the crows first begin to fly abroad and cry, the dead mother of Shuntoku came to him in a dream.

And she said to him: "Son, your affliction has been caused by the witchcraft of your wicked stepmother. Go now to the divinity of Kiyomidzu, and beseech the goddess that you may be healed."

Shuntoku arose, wondering, and took his way toward the city of Kyoto, toward the temple of Kiyomidzu.

One day, as he traveled, he went to the gate of the house of a rich man named Hagiyama, crying out loudly: "Alms! alms!"

Then a maid servant of the house, hearing the cry, came out and gave him food, and laughed aloud, saying: "Who could help laughing at the idea of trying to give anything to so comical a pilgrim?"

Shuntoku asked: "Why do you laugh? I am the son of a rich and well-famed man, Nobuyoshi of Kawachi. But because of a malediction invoked upon me by my wicked stepmother, I have become as you see me."

Then Otohime, a daughter of that family, hearing the voices, came out, and asked the maid: "Why did you laugh?"

The servant answered: "Oh, my lady, there was a blind man from Kawachi, who seemed about twenty years old, clinging to the pillar of the gate, and loudly crying, 'Alms! alms.'

"So I tried to give him some clean rice upon a tray; but when I held out the tray toward his right hand, he advanced his left; and when I held out the tray toward his left hand, he advanced his right: that was the reason I could not help laughing."

Hearing the maid explaining thus to the young lady, the blind man became angry, and said: "You have no right to despise strangers. I am the son of a rich and well-famed man in Kawachi, and I am called Shuntoku-maru."

Then the daughter of that house, Otohime, suddenly remembering him, also became quite angry, and said to the servant: "You must not laugh rudely. Laughing at others to-day, you might be laughed at yourself to-morrow."

But Otohime had been so startled that she could not help trembling a little, and, retiring to her room, she suddenly fainted away.

Then in the house all was confusion, and a doctor was summoned in great haste. But the girl, being quite unable to take any medicine, only became weaker and weaker.

Then many famous physicians were sent for; and they consulted together about Otohime; and they decided at last that her sickness had been caused only by some sudden sorrow.

So the mother said to her sick daughter "Tell me, without concealment, if you have any secret grief; and if there be anything you want, whatever it be,

I will try to get it for you."

Otohime replied: "I am very much ashamed; but I shall tell you what I wish.

"The blind man who came here the other day was the son of a rich and well-famed citizen of Kawachi, called Nobuyoshi.

"At the time of the festival of Tenjin at Kitano in Kyoto, I met that young man there, on my way to the temple; and we then exchanged letters of love, pledging ourselves to each other.

"And therefore I very much wish that I may be allowed to travel in search of him, until I find him, wherever he may be."

The mother kindly made answer: "That, indeed, will be well. If you wish for a kago, you may have one; or if you would like to have a horse, you can have one.

"You can choose any servant you like to accompany you, and I can let you have as many koban as you desire."

Otohime answered: "Neither horse nor kago do I need, nor any servant; I need only the dress of a pilgrim,—leggings and gown,—and a mendicant's wallet."

For Otohime held it her duty to set out by herself all alone, just as Shuntoku had done.

So she left home, saying farewell to her parents, with eyes full of tears: scarcely could she find voice to utter the word "good-by."

Over mountains and mountains she passed, and again over mountains; hearing only the cries of wild deer and the sound of torrent-water.

Sometimes she would lose her way; sometimes she would pursue alone a steep and difficult path; always she journeyed sorrowing.

At last she saw before her—far, far away—the pine-tree called Kawama-matsu, and the two rocks called Ota(1); and when she saw those rocks, she thought of Shuntoku with love and hope.

Hastening on, she met five or six persona going to Kumano; and she asked them: "Have you not met on your way a blind youth, about sixteen years old?"

They made answer: "No, not yet; but should we meet him anywhere, we will tell him whatever you wish."

This reply greatly disappointed Otohime; and she began to think that all her efforts to find her lover might be in vain; and she became very sad.

At last she became so sad that she resolved not to try to find him in this world anymore, but to drown herself at once in the pool of Sawara, that she might be able to meet him in a future state.

She hurried there as fast as she could. And when she reached the pond, she fixed her pilgrim's staff in the ground, and hung her outer robe on a pine-tree, and threw away her wallet, and, loosening her hair, arranged it in the style called Shimada(2).

Then, having filled her sleeves with stones, she was about to leap into the water, when there appeared suddenly before her a venerable man of seemingly not less than eighty years, robed all in white, and bearing a tablet in his hand.

And the aged man said to her: "Be not thus in haste to die, Otohime! Shuntoku whom you seek is at Kiyomidzu San: go thither and meet him."

These were, indeed, the happiest tidings she could have desired, and she became at once very happy. And she knew she had thus been saved by the august favor of her guardian deity, and that it was the god himself who had spoken to her those words.

So she cast away the stones she had put into her sleeves, and donned again the outer robe she had taken off, and rearranged her hair, and took her way in all haste to the temple of Kiyomidzu.

(1) One meaning of "Ota" in Japanese is "has met" or "have met."

(2) The simple style in which the hair of dead woman is arranged. See chapter "Of Women's Hair," in Glimpses of Unfamiliar Japan, vol. ii.

At last she reached the temple. She ascended the three lower steps, and glancing beneath a porch she saw her lover, Shuntoku, lying there asleep, covered with a straw mat; and she called to him, "Moshi! Moshi!(1)"

Shuntoku, thus being suddenly awakened, seized his staff, which was lying by his side, and cried out, "Every day the children of this neighborhood come here and annoy me, because I am blind!"

Otohime hearing these words, and feeling great sorrow, approached and laid her hands on her poor lover, and said to him:—

"I am not one of those bad, mischievous children; I am the daughter of the wealthy Hagiyama. And because I promised myself to you at the festival of Kitano Tenjin in Kyoto, I have come here to see you."

Astonished at hearing the voice of his sweet-heart, Shuntoku rose up quickly, and cried out: "Oh! are you really Otohime? It is a long time since we last met—but this is so strange! Is it not all a lie?"

And then, stroking each other, they could only cry, instead of speaking.

But presently Shuntoku, giving way to the excitement of his grief, cried out to Otohime: "A malediction has been laid upon me by my stepmother, and my appearance has been changed, as you see.

"Therefore never can I be united to you as your husband. Even as I now am, so must I remain until I fester to death.

"And so you must go back home at once, and live in happiness and splendor."

But she answered in great sorrow: "Never! Are you really in earnest? Are you truly in your right senses?

"No, no! I have disguised myself thus only because I loved you enough even to give my life for you.

"And now I will never leave you, no matter what may become of me in the future."

Shuntoku was comforted by these words; but he was also filled with pity for her, so that he wept, without being able to speak a word.

Then she said to him: "Since your wicked stepmother bewitched you only because you were rich, I am not afraid to revenge you by bewitching her also; for I, too, am the child of a rich man."

And then, with her whole heart, she spoke thus to the divinity within the temple:—"For the space of seven days and seven nights I shall remain fasting in this temple, to prove my vow; and if you have any truth and pity, I beseech you to save us.

"For so great a building as this a thatched roof is not the proper roof. I will re-roof it with feathers of little birds; and the ridge of the roof I will cover with thigh-feathers of falcons.

"This torii and these lanterns of stone are ugly: I will erect a torii of gold; and I will make a thousand lamps of gold and a thousand of silver, and every evening I will light them.

"In so large a garden as this there should be trees. I will plant a thousand hinoki, a thousand sugi, a thousand karamatsu.

"But if Shuntoku should not be healed by reason of this vow, then he and I will drown ourselves together in yonder lotos-pond.

"And after our death, taking the form of two great serpents, we will torment all who come to worship at this temple, and bar the way against pilgrims."

(1) An exclamation uttered to call the attention of another to the presence of the speaker,—from the respectful verb "to say." Our colloquial "say" does not give the proper meaning. Our "please" comes nearer to it.

Now, strange to say, on the night of the seventh day after she had vowed this vow, there came to her in a dream Kwannon-Sama who said to her:

"The prayer which you prayed I shall grant."

Forthwith Otohime awoke, and told her dream to Shuntoku, and they both wondered. They arose, and went down to the river together, and washed themselves, and worshiped the goddess.

Then, strange to say, the eyes of blind Shuntoku were fully opened, and his clear sight came back to him, and the disease passed away from him. And both wept because of the greatness of their joy.

Together they sought an inn, and there laid aside their pilgrim-dresses, and put on fresh robes, and hired kago and carriers to bear them home.

Reaching the house of his father, Shuntoku cried out: "Honored parents, I have returned to you! By virtue of the written charm upon the sacred tablet, I have been healed of my sickness, as you may see. Is all well with you, honored parents?"

And Shuntoku's father, hearing, ran out and cried: "Oh! how much troubled I have been for your sake!

"Never for one moment could I cease to think of you; but now—how glad I am to see you, and the bride you have brought with you!" And all rejoiced together.

But, on the other hand, it was very strange that the wicked stepmother at the same moment became suddenly blind, and that her fingers and her toes began to rot, so that she was in great torment.

Then the bride and the bridegroom said to that wicked stepmother:
"Lo! the leprosy has come upon you!

"We cannot keep a leper in the house of a rich man. Please to go away at once!

"We shall give you a pilgrim's gown and leggings, a rush hat, and a staff; for we have all these things ready here."

Then the wicked stepmother knew that even to save her from death it could not be helped, because she herself had done so wicked a thing before. Shuntoku and his wife were very glad; how rejoiced they were!

The stepmother prayed them to allow her only one small meal a day,—just as Shuntoku had done; but Otohime said to the stricken woman: "We cannot keep you here,—not even in the corner of an outhouse. Go away at once!"

Also Nobuyoshi said to his wicked wife: "What do you mean by remaining here? How long do you require to go?"

And he drove her out, and she could not help herself, and she went away crying, and striving to hide her face from the sight of the neighbors.

Otowaka led his blind mother by the hand; and together they went to Kyoto and to the temple of Kiyomidzu.

When they got there they ascended three of the temple steps, and knelt down, and prayed the goddess, saying: "Give us power to cast another malediction!"

But the goddess suddenly appeared before them, and said: "Were it a good thing that you pray for, I would grant your prayer; but with an evil matter I will have no more to do.

"If you must die, then die there! And after your death you shall be sent to hell, and there put into the bottom of an iron caldron to be boiled."

This is the end of the Story of Shuntoku. With a jubilant tap of the fan we finish so! Joyfully!—joyfully!—joyfully!

THE BALLAD OF OGURI-HANGWAN

To tell every word of the tale,—this is the story of Oguri-Hangwan.

I. THE BIRTH

The famed Takakura Dainagon, whose other name was Kane-ie, was so rich that he had treasure-houses in every direction.

He owned one precious stone that had power over fire, and another that had power over water.

He also had the claws of a tiger, extracted from the paws of the living animal; he had the horns of a colt; and he likewise owned even a musk-cat (jako-neko)(1).

Of all that a man might have in this world, he wanted nothing except an heir, and he had no other cause for sorrow.

A trusted servant in his house named Ikenoshoji said at last to him these words:—

"Seeing that the Buddhist deity Tamon-Ten, enshrined upon the holy mountain of Kurama, is famed for his divine favor far and near, I respectfully entreat you to go to that temple and make prayer to him; for then your wish will surely be fulfilled."

To this the master agreed, and at once began to make preparation for a journey to the temple.

As he traveled with great speed he reached the temple very soon; and there, having purified his body by pouring water over it, he prayed with all his heart for an heir.

And during three days and three nights he abstained from food of every sort. But all seemed in vain.

Wherefore the lord, despairing because of the silence of the god, resolved to perform *harakiri* in the temple, and so to defile the sacred building.

Moreover, he resolved that his spirit, after his death, should haunt the mountain of Kurama, to deter and terrify all pilgrims upon the nine-mile path of the mountain.

The delay of even one moment would have been fatal; but good Ikenoshoji came running to the place just in time, and prevented the seppuku(2).

"Oh, my lord!" the retainer cried, "you are surely too hasty in your resolve to die.

"Rather first suffer me to try my fortune, and see if I may not be able to offer up prayer for your sake with more success."

Then after having twenty-one times purified his body,—seven times washing with hot water, seven times with cold, and yet another seven times washing himself with a bundle of bamboo-grass,—he thus prayed to the god:—

"If to my lord an heir be given by the divine favor, then I vow that I will make offering of paving-blocks of bronze wherewith to pave this temple court.

"Also of lanterns of bronze to stand in rows without the temple, and of plating of pure gold and pure silver to cover all the pillars within!"

And upon the third of the three nights which he passed in prayer before the god, Tamon-Ten revealed himself to the pious Ikenoshoji and said to him:—

"Earnestly wishing to grant your petition, I sought far and near for a fitting heir,—even as far as Tenjiku (India) and Kara (China).

"But though human beings are numerous as the stars in the sky or the countless pebbles upon the shore, I was grieved that I could not find of the seed of man one heir that might well be given to your master.

"And at last, knowing not what else to do, I took away by stealth [the spirit?] of one of the eight children whose father was one of the Shi-Tenno(3), residing on the peak Ari-ari, far among the Dandoku mountains. And that child I will give to become the heir of your master."

Having thus spoken, the deity retired within the innermost shrine. Then Ikenoshoji, starting from his real dream, nine times prostrated himself before the god, and hastened to the dwelling of his master.

Erelong the wife of Takakura Dainagon found herself with child; and after the ten(4) happy months she bore a son with painless labor.

It was strange that the infant had upon his forehead, marked quite plainly and naturally, the Chinese character for "rice."

And it was yet more strange to find that in his eyes four Buddhas(5) were reflected.

Ikenoshoji and the parents rejoiced; and the name Ari-waka (Young Ari) was given the child—after the name of the mountain Ari-ari —on the third day after the birth.

(1)"Musk-rat" is the translation given by some dictionaries. "Musk-deer" was suggested by my translator. But as some mythological animal is evidently meant, I thought it better to translate the word literally.

(2) The Chinese term for harakiri. It is thought to be the more refined word.

(3) Shi-Tenno: the Four Deva Kings of Buddhism, who guard the Four Quarters of the World.

(4) That is, ten by the ancient native manner of reckoning time.

(5) Shitai-no-mi-Hotoke: literally, a four-bodied-august Buddha. The image in the eye is called the Buddha: the idea here expressed seems to be that the eyes of the child reflected four instead of two images. Children of supernatural beings were popularly said to have double pupils. But I am giving only a popular explanation of the term.

II. THE BANISHMENT

Very quickly the child grew; and when he became fifteen, the reigning Emperor gave him the name and title of Oguri-Hangwan Kane-uji.

When he reached manhood his father resolved to get him a bride.

So the Dainagon looked upon all the daughters of the ministers and high officials, but he found none that he thought worthy to become the wife of his son.

But the young Hangwan, learning that he himself had been a gift to his parents from Tamon-Ten, resolved to pray to that deity for a spouse; and he hastened to the temple of the divinity, accompanied by Ikenoshoji.

There they washed their hands and rinsed their mouths, and remained three nights without sleep, passing all the time in religious exercises.

But as they had no companions, the young prince at last felt very lonesome, and began to play on his flute, made of the root of the bamboo.

Seemingly charmed by these sweet sounds, the great serpent that lived in the temple pond came to the entrance of the temple,—transforming its fearful shape into the likeness of a lovely female attendant of the Imperial Court,—and fondly listened to the melody.

Then Kane-uji thought he saw before him the very lady he desired for a wife. And thinking also that she was the one chosen for him by the deity, he placed the beautiful being in a palanquin and returned to his home.

But no sooner had this happened than a fearful storm burst upon the capital, followed by a great flood; and the flood and the storm both lasted for seven days and seven nights.

The Emperor was troubled greatly by these omens; and he sent for the astrologers, that they might explain the causes thereof.

They said in answer to the questions asked of them that the terrible weather was caused only by the anger of the male serpent, seeking vengeance for the loss of its mate,—which was none other than the fair woman that Kane-uji had brought back with him.

Whereupon the Emperor commanded that Kane-uji should be banished to the province of Hitachi, and that the transformed female serpent should at once be taken back to the pond upon the mountain of Kurama.

And being thus compelled by imperial order to depart, Kane-uji went away to the province of Hitachi, followed only by his faithful retainer, Ikenoshoji.

III. THE EXCHANGE OF LETTERS

Only a little while after the banishment of Kane-uji, a traveling merchant, seeking to sell his wares, visited the house of the exiled prince at Hitachi.

And being asked by the Hangwan where he lived, the merchant made answer, saying:—"I live in Kyoto, in the street called Muromachi, and my name is Goto Sayemon.

"My stock consists of goods of one thousand and eight different kinds which I send to China, of one thousand and eight kinds which I send to India, and yet another thousand and eight kinds which I sell only in Japan.

"So that my whole stock consists of three thousand and twenty-four different kinds of goods.

"Concerning the countries to which I have already been, I may answer that I made three voyages to India and three to China and this is my seventh journey to this part of Japan."

Having heard these things, Oguri-Hangwan asked the merchant whether he knew of any young girl who would make a worthy wife, since he, the prince, being still unmarried, desired to find such a girl.

Then said Sayemon: "In the province of Sagami, to the west of us, there lives a rich man called Tokoyama Choja, who has eight sons.

"Long he lamented that he had no daughter, and he long prayed for a daughter to the August Sun.

"And a daughter was given him; and after her birth, her parents thought it behoved them to give her a higher rank than their own, because her birth had come to pass through the divine influence of the August Heaven-Shining Deity; so they built for her a separate dwelling.

"She is, in very truth, superior to all other Japanese women; nor can I think of any other person in every manner worthy of you."

This story much pleased Kane-uji; and he at once asked Sayemon to act the part of match-maker(1) for him; and Sayemon promised to do everything in his power to fulfill the wish of the Hangwan.

Then Kane-uji called for inkstone and writing-brush, and wrote a love-letter, and tied it up with such a knot as love-letters are tied with.

And he gave it to the merchant to be delivered to the lady; and he gave him also, in reward for his services, one hundred golden ryo.

Sayemon again and again prostrated himself in thanks; and he put the letter into the box which he always carried with him. And then he lifted the box upon his back, and bade the prince fare-well.

Now, although the journey from Hitachi to Sagami is commonly a journey of seven days, the merchant arrived there at noon upon the third day, having traveled in all haste, night and day together, without stopping.

And he went to the building called Inui-no-Goshyo, which had been built by the rich Yokoyama for the sake of his only daughter, Terute-Hime, in the district of Soba, in the province of Sagami; and he asked permission to enter therein.

But the stern gate-keepers bade him go away, announcing that the dwelling was the dwelling of Terute-Hime, daughter of the famed Choja Yokoyama, and that no person of the male sex whosoever could be permitted to enter; and furthermore, that guards had been appointed to guard the palace—ten by night and ten by day—with extreme caution and severity.

But the merchant told the gate-keepers that he was Goto Sayemon, of the street called Muromachi, in the city of Kyoto; that he was a well-famed merchant there, and was by the people called Sendanya; that he had thrice been to India and thrice to China, and was now upon his seventh return journey to the great country of the Rising Sun.

And he said also to them: "Into all the palaces of Nihon, save this one only, I have been freely admitted; so I shall be deeply grateful to you if you permit me to enter."

Thus saying, he produced many rolls of silk, and presented them to the gate-keepers; and their cupidity made them blind; and the merchant, without more difficulty, entered, rejoicing.

Through the great outer gate he passed, and over a bridge, and then found himself in front of the chambers of the female attendants of the superior class.

And he called out with a very loud voice: "O my ladies, all things that you may require I have here with me!

"I have all *jorogata-no-meshi-dogu*; I have hair-combs and needles and tweezers; I have *tategami,* and combs of silver, and *kamoji* from Nagasaki, and even all kinds of Chinese mirrors!"

Whereupon the ladies, delighted with the idea of seeing these things, suffered the merchant to enter their apartment, which he presently made to look like a shop for the sale of female toilet articles.

(1) Nakodo. The profession of nakodo exists; but any person who arranges marriages for a consideration is for the time being called the nakodo.

But while making bargains and selling very quickly, Sayemon did not lose the good chance offered him; and taking from his box the love-letter which had been confided to him, he said to the ladies:—

"This letter, if I remember rightly, I picked up in some town in Hitachi, and I shall be very glad if you will accept it,—either to use it for a model if it be written beautifully, or to laugh at if it prove to have been written awkwardly."

Then the chief among the maids, receiving the letter, tried to read the writing upon the envelope: *"Tsuki ni hoshi—ame ni arare ga—kori kana,"*—

Which signified, "Moon and stars—rain and hail—make ice." But she could not read the riddle of the mysterious words.

The other ladies, who were also unable to guess the meaning of the words, could not but laugh; and they laughed so shrilly that the Princess Terute heard, and came among them, fully robed, and wearing a veil over her night-black hair.

And the bamboo-screen having been rolled up before her, Terute-Hime asked: "What is the cause of all this laughing? If there be anything amusing, I wish that you will let me share in the amusement."

The maids then answered, saying: "We were laughing only at our being unable to read a letter which this merchant from the capital says that he picked up in some street. And here is the letter: even the address upon it is a riddle to us."

And the letter, having been laid upon an open crimson fan, was properly presented to the princess, who received it, and admired the beauty of the writing, and said:—

"Never have I seen so beautiful a hand as this: it is like the writing of Kobodaishi himself, or of Monju Bosatsu.

"Perhaps the writer is one of those princes of the Ichijo, or Nijo, or Sanjo families, all famed for their skill in writing.

"Or, if this guess of mine be wrong, then I should say that these characters have certainly been written by Oguri-Hangwan Kane-uji, now so famed in the province of Hitachi…. I shall read the letter for you."

Then the envelope was removed; and the first phrase she read was *Fuji no yama* (the Mountain of Fuji), which she interpreted as signifying loftiness of rank. And then she met with such phrases as these:—

Kiyomidzu kosaka (the name of a place); *arare ni ozasa* (hail on the leaves of the bamboo-grass); *itaya ni arare* (hail following upon a wooden roof);

Tamato ni kori (ice in the sleeve); *nonaka ni shimidzu* (pure water running through a moor); *koike ni makomo* (rushes in a little pond);

Inoba ni tsuyu (dew on the leaves of the taro); *shakunaga obi* (a very long girdle); *shika ni momiji* (deer and maple-trees);

Futamata-gawa (a forked river); *hoso tanigawa-ni marukibashi* (a round log laid over a little stream for a bridge); *tsurunashi yumi ni hanuki dori* (a stringless bow, and a wingless bird).

And then she understood that the characters signified:—

Maireba au—they would meet, for he would call upon her. *Arare nai*—then they would not be separated. *Korobi au*—they would repose together.

And the meaning of the rest was thus:—

"This letter should be opened within the sleeve, so that others may know nothing of it. Keep the secret in your own bosom.

"You must yield to me even as the rush bends to the wind. I am earnest to serve you in all things.

"We shall surely be united at last, whatever chance may separate us at the beginning. I wish for you even as the stag for its mate in the autumn.

"Even though long kept apart we shall meet, as meet the waters of a river divided in its upper course into two branches.

"Divine, I pray you, the meaning of this letter, and preserve it. I hope for a fortunate answer. Thinking of Terute-Hime, I feel as though I could fly."

And the Princess Terute found at the end of the letter the name of him who wrote it,—Oguri-Hangwan Kane-uji himself,—together with her own name, as being written to her.

Then she felt greatly troubled, because she had not at first supposed that the letter was addressed to her, and had, without thinking, read it aloud to the female attendants.

For she well knew that her father would quickly kill her in a most cruel manner, should the iron-hearted Choja(1) come to know the truth.

Wherefore, through fear of being mingled with the earth of the moor Uwanogahara,—fitting place for a father in wrath to slay his daughter,—she set the end of the letter between her teeth, and rent it to pieces, and withdrew to the inner apartment.

(1) Choja is not a proper name: it signifies really a wealthy man only, like the French terms "un richard," "un riche." But it is used almost like a proper name in the country still; the richest man in the place, usually a person of influence, being often referred to as "the Choja."

But the merchant, knowing that he could not go back to Hitachi without bearing some reply, resolved to obtain one by cunning.

Wherefore he hurried after the princess even into her innermost apartment, without so much as waiting to remove his sandals, and he cried out loudly:—"Oh, my princess! I have been taught that written characters were invented in India by Monju Bosatsu, and in Japan by Kobodaishi.

"And is it not like tearing the hands of Kobodaishi, thus to tear a letter written with characters?

"Know you not that a woman is less pure than a man? Wherefore, then, do you, born a woman, thus presume to tear a letter?

"Now, if you refuse to write a reply, I shall call upon all the gods; I shall announce to them this unwomanly act, and I shall invoke their malediction upon you!"

And with these words he took from the box which he always carried with him a Buddhist rosary; and he began to twist it about with an awful appearance of anger.

Then the Princess Terute, terrified and grieved, prayed him to cease his invocations, and promised that she would write an answer at once.

So her answer was quickly written, and given to the merchant, who was overjoyed by his success, and speedily departed for Hitachi, carrying his box upon his back.

IV. HOW KANE-UJI BECAME A BRIDEGROOM WITHOUT HIS FATHER-IN-LAW'S CONSENT

Traveling with great speed, the nakodo quickly arrived at the dwelling of the Hangwan, and gave the letter to the master, who removed the cover with hands that trembled for joy.

Very, very short the answer was,—only these words: *Oki naka bune*, "a boat floating in the offing."

But Kane-uji guessed the meaning to be: "As fortunes and misfortunes are common to all, be not afraid, and try to come unseen."

Therewith he summoned Ikenoshoji, and bade him make all needful preparation for a rapid journey. Goto Sayemon consented to serve as guide.

He accompanied them; and when they reached the district of Soba, and were approaching the house of the princess, the guide said to the prince:—

"That house before us, with the black gate, is the dwelling of the far-famed Yokoyama Choja; and that other house, to the northward of it, having a red gate, is the residence of the flower-fair Terute.

"Be prudent in all things, and you will succeed." And with these words, the guide disappeared.

Accompanied by his faithful retainer, the Hangwan approached the red gate.

Both attempted to enter, when the gate-keeper sought to prevent them; declaring they were much too bold to seek to enter the dwelling of Terute-Hime, only daughter of the renowned Yokoyama Choja,—the sacred child begotten through the favor of the deity of the Sun.

"You do but right to speak thus," the retainer made reply. "But you must learn that we are officers from the city in search of a fugitive.

"And it is just because all males are prohibited from entering this dwelling that a search therein must be made."

Then the guards, amazed, suffered them to pass, and saw the supposed officers of justice enter the court, and many of the ladies in waiting come forth to welcome them as guests.

And the Lady Terute, marvelously pleased by the coming of the writer of that love-letter, appeared before her wooer, robed in her robes of ceremony, with a veil about her shoulders.

Kane-uji was also much delighted at being thus welcomed by the beautiful maiden. And the wedding ceremony was at once performed, to the great joy of both, and was followed by a great wine feast.

So great was the mirth, and so joyful were all, that the followers of the prince and the maids of the princess danced together, and together made music.

And Oguri-Hangwan himself produced his flute, made of the root of a bamboo, and began to play upon it sweetly.

Then the father of Terute, hearing all this joyous din in the house of his daughter, wondered greatly what the cause might be.

But when he had been told how the Hangwan had become the bridegroom of his daughter without his consent, the Choja grew wondrous angry, and in secret devised a scheme of revenge.

V. THE POISONING

The next day Yokoyama sent to Prince Kane-uji a message, inviting him to come to his house, there to perform the wine-drinking ceremony of greeting each other as father-in-law and son-in-law.

Then the Princess Terute sought to dissuade the Hangwan from going there, because she had dreamed in the night a dream of ill omen.

But the Hangwan, making light of her fears, went boldly to the dwelling of the Choja, followed by his young retainers. Then Yokoyama Choja, rejoicing, caused many dishes to be prepared, containing all delicacies furnished by the mountains and the sea(1), and well entertained the Hangwan.

At last, when the wine-drinking began to flag, Yokoyama uttered the wish that his guest, the lord Kane-uji, would also furnish some entertainment(2).

"And what shall it be?" the Hangwan asked.

"Truly," replied the Choja, "I am desirous to see you show your great skill in riding."

"Then I shall ride," the prince made answer. And presently the horse called Onikage(3) was led out.

That horse was so fierce that he did not seem to be a real horse, but rather a demon or a dragon, so that few dared even to approach him.

But the Prince Hangwan Kane-uji at once loosened the chain by which the horse was fastened, and rode upon him with wondrous ease.

In spite of his fierceness, Onikage found himself obliged to do everything which his rider wished. All present, Yokoyama and the others, could not speak for astonishment.

But soon the Choja, taking and setting up a six-folding screen, asked to see the prince ride his steed upon the upper edge of the screen.

The lord Oguri, consenting, rode upon the top of the screen; and then he rode along the top of an upright shoji frame.

Then a chessboard being set out, he rode upon it, making the horse rightly set his hoof upon the squares of the chessboard as he rode.

And, lastly, he made the steed balance himself upon the frame of an andon(4).

Then Yokoyama was at a loss what to do, and he could only say, bowing low to the prince:

"Truly I am grateful for your entertainment; I am very much delighted."

And the lord Oguri, having attached Onikage to a cherry-tree in the garden, reentered the apartment.

But Saburo, the third son of the house, having persuaded his father to kill the Hangwan with poisoned wine, urged the prince to drink sake with which there had been mingled the venom of a blue centipede and of a blue lizard, and foul water that had long stood in the hollow joint of a bamboo.

And the Hangwan and his followers, not suspecting the wine had been poisoned, drank the whole.

Sad to say, the poison entered into their viscera and their intestines; and all their bones burst asunder by reason of the violence of that poison.

(1) Or, "with all strange flavors of mountain and sea."

(2) The word is really sakana, "fish." It has always been the rule to serve fish with sake; and gradually the word "fish" became used for any entertainment given during the wine-party by guests, such as songs, dances, etc.

(3) Literally, "Demon-deer-hair." The term "deer-hair" refers to color. A less exact translation of the original characters would be "the demon chestnut". Kage, "deer-color" also means "chestnut." A chestnut horse is Kage-no-uma.

(4) A large portable lantern, having a wooden frame and paper sides. There are andon of many forms, some remarkably beautiful.

Their lives passed from them quickly as dew in the morning from the grass.

And Saburo and his father buried their corpses in the moor Uwanogahara.

VI. CAST ADRIFT

The cruel Yokoyama thought that it would not do to suffer his daughter to live, after he had thus killed her husband. Therefore he felt obliged to order his faithful servants, Onio and Oniji, (1) who were brothers, to take her far out into the sea of Sagami, and to drown her there.

And the two brothers, knowing their master was too stony-hearted to be persuaded otherwise, could do nothing but obey. So they went to the unhappy lady, and told her the purpose for which they had been sent.

Terute-Hime was so astonished by her father's cruel decision that at first she thought all this was a dream, from which she earnestly prayed to be awakened.

After a while she said: "Never in my whole life have I knowingly committed any crime…. But whatever happens to my own body, I am more anxious than I can say to learn what became of my husband after he visited my father's house."

"Our master," answered the two brothers, "becoming very angry at learning that you two had been wedded without his lawful permission, poisoned the young prince, according to a plan devised by your brother Saburo."

Then Terute, more and more astonished, invoked, with just cause, a malediction upon her father for his cruelty.

But she was not even allowed time to lament her fate; for Onio and his brother at once removed her garments, and put her naked body into a roll of rush matting.

When this piteous package was carried out of the house at night, the princess and her waiting-maids bade each other their last farewells, with sobs and cries of grief.

(1) Onio, "the king of devils," Oniji, "the next greatest devil."

The brothers Onio and Oniji then rowed far out to sea with their pitiful burden. But when they found themselves alone, then Oniji said to Onio that it were better they should try to save their young mistress.

To this the elder brother at once agreed without difficulty; and both began to think of some plan to save her.

Just at the same time an empty canoe came near them, drifting with the sea-current.

At once the lady was placed in it; and the brothers, exclaiming, "That indeed was a fortunate happening," bade their mistress farewell, and rowed back to their master.

VII. THE LADY YORIHIME

The canoe bearing poor Terute was tossed about by the waves for seven days and seven nights, during which time there was much wind and rain. And at last it was discovered by some fishermen who were fishing near Nawoye.

But they thought that the beautiful woman was certainly the spirit that had caused the long storm of many days; and Terute might have been killed by their oars, had not one of the men of Nawoye taken her under his protection.

Now this man, whose name was Murakimi Dayu, resolved to adopt the princess as his daughter as he had no child of his own to be his heir.

So he took her to his home, and named her Yorihime, and treated her so kindly that his wife grew jealous of the adopted daughter, and therefore was often cruel to her when the husband was absent.

But being still more angered to find that Yorihime would not go away of her own accord, the evil-hearted woman began to devise some means of getting rid of her forever.

Just at that time the ship of a kidnapper happened to cast anchor in the harbor. Needless to say that Yorihime was secretly sold to this dealer in human flesh.

VIII. BECOMING A SERVANT

After this misfortune, the unhappy princess passed from one master to another as many as seventy-five times. Her last purchaser was one Yorodzuya Chobei, well known as the keeper of a large joroya(1) in the province of Mino.

When Terute-Hime was first brought before this new master, she spoke meekly to him, and begged him to excuse her ignorance of all refinements and of deportment. And Chobei then asked her to tell him all about herself, her native place, and her family. But Terute-Hime thought it would not be wise to mention even the name of her native province, lest she might possibly be forced to speak of the poisoning of her husband by her own father.

So she resolved to answer only that she was born in Hitachi; feeling a sad pleasure in saying that she belonged to the same province in which the lord Hangwan, her lover, used to live.

"I was born," she said, "in the province of Hitachi; but I am of too low birth to have a family name. Therefore may I beseech you to bestow some suitable name upon me?"

Then Terute-Hime was named Kohagi of Hitachi, and she was told that she would have to serve her master very faithfully in his business.

But this order she refused to obey, and said that she would perform with pleasure any work given her to do, however mean or hard, but that she would never follow the business of a joro.

"Then," cried Chobei in anger, "your daily tasks shall be these:—

"To feed all the horses, one hundred in number, that are kept in the stables, and to wait upon all other persons in the house when they take their meals.

"To dress the hair of the thirty-six joro belonging to this house, dressing the hair of each in the style that best becomes her; and also to fill seven boxes with threads of twisted hemp.

"Also to make the fire daily in seven furnaces, and to draw water from a spring in the mountains, half a mile from here."

Terute knew that neither she nor any other being alive could possibly fulfill all the tasks thus laid upon her by this cruel master; and she wept over her misfortune.

But she soon felt that to weep could avail her nothing. So wiping away her tears, she bravely resolved to try what she could do, and then putting on an apron, and tying back her sleeves, she set to work feeding the horses.

The great mercy of the gods cannot be understood; but it is certain that as she fed the first horse, all the others, through divine influence, were fully fed at the same time.

And the same wonderful thing happened when she waited upon the people of the house at mealtime, and when she dressed the hair of the girls, and when she twisted the threads of hemp, and when she went to kindle the fire in the furnaces.

But saddest of all it was to see Terute-Hime bearing the water-buckets upon her shoulders, taking her way to the distant spring to draw water.

After a single week the effects of the bath caused the eyes, nose, ears, and mouth to reappear; after fourteen days all the limbs had been fully reformed;

And after one-and-twenty days the nameless shape was completely transformed into the real Oguri-Hangwan Kane-uji, perfect and handsome as he had been in other years.

When this marvelous change had been effected, Kane-uji looked all about him, and wondered much when and how he had been brought to that strange place.

But through the august influence of the god of Kumano things were so ordained that the revived prince could return safely to his home at Nijo in Kyoto, where his parents, the lord Kane-ie and his spouse, welcomed him with great joy.

Then the august Emperor, hearing all that had happened, thought it a wonderful thing that one of his subjects, after having been dead three years, should have thus revived.

And not only did he gladly pardon the fault for which the Hangwan had been banished, but further appointed him to be lord ruler of the three provinces, Hitachi, Sagami, and Mino.

XI. THE INTERVIEW

One day Oguri-Hangwan left his residence to make a journey of inspection through the provinces of which he had been appointed ruler. And reaching Mino, he resolved to visit Kohagi of Hitachi, and to utter his thanks to her for her exceeding goodness.

Therefore he lodged at the house of Yorodzuya, where he was conducted to the finest of all the guest-chambers, which was made beautiful with screens of gold, with Chinese carpets, with Indian hangings, and with other precious things of great cost.

When the lord ordered Kohagi of Hitachi to be summoned to his presence, he was answered that she was only one of the lowest menials, and too dirty to appear before him. But he paid no heed to these words, only commanding that she should come at once, no matter how dirty she might be.

Therefore, much against her will, Kohagi was obliged to appear before the lord, whom she at first beheld through a screen, and saw that he was so much like the Hangwan that she was greatly startled.

Oguri then asked her to tell him her real name; but Kohagi refused, saying: "If I may not serve my lord with wine, except on condition of telling my real name, then I can only leave the presence of my lord."

But as she was about to go, the Hangwan called to her: "Nay, stop a little while. I have a good reason to ask your name, because I am in truth that very *gaki-ami* whom you so kindly drew last year to Otsu in a cart."

And with these words he produced the wooden tablet upon which Kohagi had written.

Then she was greatly moved, and said: "I am very happy to see you thus recovered. And now I shall gladly tell you all my history; hoping only that you, my lord, will tell me something of that ghostly world from which you have come back, and in which my husband, alas, now dwells.

"I was born (it hurts my heart to speak of former times!) the only daughter of Yokoyama Choja, who dwelt in the district of Soba, in the province of Sagami, and my name was Terute-Hime.

"I remember too well, alas! having been wedded, three years ago, to a famous person of rank, whose name was Oguri-Hangwan Kane-uji, who used to live in the province of Hitachi. But my husband was poisoned by my father at the instigation of his own third son, Saburo.

"I myself was condemned by him to be drowned in the sea of Sagami. And I owe my present existence to the faithful servants of my father, Onio and Oniji."

Then the lord Hangwan said, "You see here before you, Terute, your husband, Kane-uji. Although killed together with my followers, I had been destined to live in this world many years longer.

"By the learned priest of Fujisawa temple I was saved, and, being provided with a cart, I was drawn by many kind persons to the hot springs of Kumano, where I was restored to my former health and shape. And now I have been appointed lord ruler of the three provinces, and can have all things that I desire."

Hearing this tale, Terute could scarcely believe it was not all a dream, and she wept for joy. Then she said: "Ah! since last I saw you, what hardships have I not passed through!

"For seven days and seven nights I was tossed about upon the sea in a canoe; then I was in a great danger in the bay of Nawoye, and was saved by a kind man called Murakami Deyu.

"And after that I was sold and bought seventy-five times; and the last time I was brought here, where I have been made to suffer all kinds of hardship only because I refused to become a joro. That is why you now see me in so wretched a condition."

Very angry was Kane-uji to hear of the cruel conduct of the inhuman Chobei, and desired to kill him at once.

But Terute besought her husband to spare the man's life, and so fulfilled the promise she had long before made to Chobei,—that she would give even her own life, if necessary, for her master and mistress, on condition of being allowed five days' freedom to draw the cart of the *gaki-ami*.

And for this Chobei was really grateful; and in compensation he presented the Hangwan with the hundred horses from his stable, and gave to Terute the thirty-six servants belonging to his house.

And then Terute-Hime, appropriately attired, went away with the Prince Kane-uji; and, they began their journey to Sagami with hearts full of joy.

XII. THE VENGEANCE

This is the district of Soba, in the province of Sagami, the native land of Terute: how many beautiful and how many sorrowful thoughts does it recall to their minds!

And here also are Yokoyama and his son, who killed Lord Ogiri with poison.

So Saburo, the third son, being led to the moor called Totsuka-no-hara, was there punished.

But Yokoyama Choja, wicked as he had been, was not punished; because parents, however bad, must be for their children always like the sun and moon. And hearing this order, Yokoyama repented very greatly for that which he had done.

Qnio and Oniji, the brothers, were rewarded with many gifts for having saved the Princess Terute off the coast of Sagami.

Thus those who were good prospered, and the bad were brought to destruction.

Fortunate and happy, Oguri-Sama and Terute-Hime together returned to Miako, to dwell in the residence at Nijo, and their union was beautiful as the blossoming of spring.

Fortunate! Fortunate!

THE BALLAD OF O-SHICHI, THE DAUGHTER OF THE YAOYA (1)

In autumn the deer are lured within reach of the hunters by the sounds of the flute, which resemble the sounds of the voices of their mates, and so are killed.

Almost in like manner, one of the five most beautiful girls in Yedo, whose comely faces charmed all the capital even as the spring-blossoming of cherry-trees, cast away her life in the moment of blindness caused by love.

When, having done a foolish thing, she was brought before the mayor of the city of Yedo, that high official questioned the young criminal, asking:

"Are you not O-Shichi, the daughter of the yaoya? And being so young, how came you to commit such a dreadful crime as incendiarism?"

Then O-Shichi, weeping and wringing her hands, made this answer: "Indeed, that is the only crime I ever committed; and I had no extraordinary reason for it but this:—

"Once before, when there had been a great fire,—so great a fire that nearly all Yedo was consumed,—our house also was burned down. And we three,—my parents and I,—knowing no otherwhere to go, took shelter in a Buddhist temple, to remain there until our house could be rebuilt.

"Surely the destiny that draws two young persons to each other is hard to understand!… In that temple there was a young acolyte, and love grew up between us.

"In secret we met together, and promised never to forsake each other; and we pledged ourselves to each other by sucking blood from small cuts we made in our little fingers, and by exchanging written vows that we should love each other forever.

"Before our pillows had yet become fixed(2), our new house in Hongo was built and made ready for us.

"But from that day when I bade a sad farewell to Kichiza-Sama, to whom I had pledged myself for the time of two existences, never was my heart consoled by even one letter from the acolyte.

"Alone in my bed at night, I used to think and think, and at last in a dream there came to me the dreadful idea of setting fire to the house, as the only means of again being able to meet my beautiful lover.

"Then, one evening, I got a bundle of dry rushes, and placed inside it some pieces of live charcoal, and I secretly put the bundle into a shed at the back of the house.

"A fire broke out, and there was a great tumult, and I was arrested and brought here—oh! how dreadful it was!

"I will never, never commit such a fault again. But whatever happen, oh, pray save me, my Bugyo(3)! Oh, pray take pity on me!"

Ah! the simple apology!... But what was her age? Not twelve? not thirteen? not fourteen? Fifteen comes after fourteen. Alas! she was fifteen, and could not be saved!

Therefore O-Shichi was sentenced according to the law. But first she was bound with strong cords, and was for seven days exposed to public view on the bridge called Nihonbashi. Ah! what a piteous sight it was!

Her aunts and cousins, even Bekurai and Kakusuke, the house servants, had often to wring their sleeves, so wet were their sleeves with tears.

But, because the crime could not be forgiven, O-Shichi was bound to four posts, and fuel was kindled, and the fire rose up!... And poor O-Shichi in the midst of that fire!

Even so the insects of summer fly to the flame.

(1) Yaoya, a seller of vegetables.

(2) This curious expression has its origin in the Japanese saying that lovers "exchange pillows." In the dark, the little Japanese wooden pillows might easily be exchanged by mistake. "While the pillows, were yet not

definite or fixed" would mean, therefore, while the two lovers were still in the habit of seeking each other secretly at night.

(3) Governor or local chief. The Bugyo of old days often acted as judge.